PUT DOWN
AND RIPPED OFF
The American Woman
and the Beauty Cult

PUT DOWN AND RIPPED OFF

The American Woman and the Beauty Cult

NORA SCOTT KINZER

Thomas Y. Crowell Company · New York · Established 1834

Part of chapter 4 originally appeared in Saturday Evening Post, *December 1974, under the title "Beast and the Beauty Parlor" and is reprinted with permission. Part of chapter 6 originally appeared in* Psychology Today, *August 1973, under the title "Soapy Sin in the Afternoon." Reprinted by permission of* Psychology Today *magazine. Copyright © 1973 Ziff-Davis Publishing Company.*

Designed by Joy Chu

Manufactured in the United States of America

Library of Congress Cataloging in Publication Data

Kinzer, Nora Scott.   Put down and ripped off.

Includes index.
1. Women—United States—Social conditions.
2. Women as consumers—United States.
3. Beauty, Personal.
4. Women—Health and hygiene—United States—Sociological aspects. I. Title.
HQ1426.K56   301.41′2′0973   77-3619
ISBN 0-690-01243-8

10 9 8 7 6 5 4 3 2 1

For the five men in my life
who constantly remind me
of my fallibility.

Donald
Andrew
John
Peter
Patrick

Contents

PUT DOWN
AND RIPPED OFF
The American Woman
and the Beauty Cult

1 Mired in the Beauty Trap

I was a well-brought-up bourgeois middle-class little girl with all the homilies and traditions of being a middle-class American child. The only problem was all the things I learned about and cared about didn't make sense. They still don't, but I hearken to their call.

My mother used to tell me that it wasn't what a person looked like that mattered as long as that person had a "beautiful soul." But reality was another matter: My childhood preparations for Sunday school involved shiny, well-brushed shoes, white stockings, white gloves, flowered hat, and stiffly starched petticoat. God, cleanliness, fashion, and the latest fads were all intertwined. Easter was the day when God and *Vogue* magazine met. My mother and I always had new hats, if not new outfits, and my father managed at least a new tie—after he had paid our bills.

So it was off to Sunday school with white gloves; later it was off to the prom with a tulle strapless; and finally, off to cocktail parties with the simple little black dress. I learned quickly that cute little girls in nice pinafores and sexy young women in simple black dresses were inordinately more socially acceptable than plain Janes with beautiful souls. My life was ruled by fads, fashions, crazes, and a certain amount of craziness.

Craziness meant hysterics and tears when a pimple appeared, worry about an extra ten pounds in the wrong places, and a frenetic search through boutiques and department stores for the perfect scarf to match an exquisite blouse. But I didn't think I was crazy. If I was loony, so were (and are) most of my friends. We all found ourselves primping before mirrors, frizzing our hair under hot dryers, shoving our feet into pointy-toed shoes, and generally enjoying our self-inflicted torture. Why not? We are the latest descendants of thousands of years of primping, combing, dieting, tattooing, and body painting. We are the willing victims of a consumer society! We are the women caught in the iron-meshed spider web of mass advertising. We are made ashamed of bodies. We seek to become something else. If the current *you* is not beautiful or thin, blond or tweezed according to the latest fashion dictates, then painting, starving, dyeing, and tweezing will produce a new and more appropriate *you*.

The American female is always in a state of becoming. She is an unfinished, incomplete, never-perfected product.

No matter what she buys, wears, or looks like, there is always something missing. If her skirt is short, the magazines tell her it should be long. If her hair is brown, the TV advertisements tell her, "Blondes have more fun." If she bleaches her hair and buys the latest fad clothes, the next message she hears is that "the natural look is in." She is either too fat or too thin. She should have large breasts, but only the young and firm can go braless. However, since excessively large breasts are a liability, surgery can pare off any excess. Ms. America resorts to chicanery, deception, surgery, fad diets, starvation, fat farms, *anything,* in order to attain the unattainable. In short, she is constantly miserable and continuously in a feverish rush to be *au courant.*

Promised beauty, allure, adulation, and fortune, she guilelessly buys whatever product is hawked over the air or in the pages of her favorite publication. She joins diet clubs; she bumps, starves, groans, and rumbles; exercise salons take her money: all to no avail.

She never attains nirvana. She never becomes the soigné, chic fashion plate. She is always Mrs. Lump-Lump in her Robert Hall imitation Courrèges. She may impress the checkout girl at the grocery store, but not the country-club set. No wonder then that so many high-school-educated, white American housewives gobble tranquilizers and swill booze—in between eating far too many calories. Wouldn't you? Or do you?

Miracles are promised to each and every American woman. Buy me and I will transform you! Enroll in my school and you will become charming! Eat me and I will make you effortlessly and magically thin! Wear me and I will grind away your bumps and lumps! In this unreal land, enchantment reigns supreme.

What woman thumbing through a fashion magazine has not imagined herself fifteen—or fifty—pounds thinner, and a model herself? What American housewife has not gone to a hairdresser clutching a picture of Raquel Welch, convinced that with a similar hair style the movie-star ambience will also miraculously follow? Who has not read the gory stories in pulp magazines and felt a vicarious shiver of excitement or a sense of moral superiority to the heroines ensnared in turpitude?

The answer is—none of us. Anyway that's what I learned from some long years of pondering the inner meaning of beauty and the snares of a peculiar woman's culture, and I will publicly admit that I'm mired in the beauty trap.

There *is* a strange, weird, wonderful, and lunatic woman's culture in the United States. But, what's more interesting is that very few social scientists admit that such a culture exists. I spent long years in graduate school learning about exotic tribes like the Ashanti, Yoruba, and Bushman. I pored over anthropology texts about Egyptian dress and style and studied about norms and rules of behavior of alien tribes. But when I suggested that perhaps hairdressers and fat farms were interesting manifestations of American culture, my professors dismissed me with sneers and snarls. I spent endless hours in libraries studying the origins of folk literature of Mexico and how Shakespeare evolved from traveling troubadours of the Middle Ages. But when I asked if perhaps soap operas were not the folk theater of the modern-day United States, their scorn and derision increased.

Because, of course, Sociology had decided what were intellectually acceptable topics. Go-go dancers, perverts, disturbed children, damaged families, alcoholics, and drug addicts were acceptable intellectual subjects worthy of dissertations, books, and jargon-laden professional articles. But hairdressers and soap operas were not. Anyway, besides all that, these professors were men, and the woman's world and woman's culture interested them not. Yet, as a woman, as a sociologist, as a product of thousands of years of woman's culture, and as a nice middle-class lady, I had my secret vices.

My male colleagues and erstwhile professors couldn't possibly understand woman's culture. Like many girls in the 1940's, I had been weaned on *Our Gal Sunday* and *Helen Trent.* In grade school over my lunchtime sandwiches I worried "whether an orphan girl from a little mining town in the West could find happiness as the wife of England's richest, most handsome lord." And I wondered if indeed "a woman could find happiness and love at thirty-six and even beyond."

So some twenty years later, on those afternoons when I wasn't teaching, I graded papers at home and watched my favorite soap operas. My friends began to treat my vice with the same kind of attitude they showed to a secret drinker. No one dared telephone me when *The Doctors* was on and woe betide anyone who tried to communicate with me during *Secret Shadows*! I had a nagging feeling that maybe

I was a little strange but consoled myself with the fact that there were at least three million other nuts like me in the United States. I started delving into soap-opera culture and found that the audience indeed was predominantly house-wives and that soap operas were the financial backbone of all three networks.

So to justify my moral turpitude I dissected soap operas in a *Psychology Today* article that met with yowls from outraged fans and critical acclaim from the anthropologists. Erich Fromm had an article in the same issue and the mail for my ephemeral piece outweighed his pound for pound. My career as a popular-culture freak had taken an upswing. While I became intellectually acceptable and could justify my addiction, the truth of the matter still remains—I enjoy the soaps.

There's where my ambivalence lies. I may look at the world with the jaundiced eye of a social scientist but this is my own world. I am part of the woman's culture and can neither deride nor sneer nor even be objective because I am a creature of this very world. There are appropriate rules of behavior and dress that I would never dare flout. Why? Because my mother, grandmother, and great-grandmother, aunts, female cousins, and assorted great-aunts taught me these rules and instilled in me a sense of shame and guilt were they to be broken.

And my guilt reached an all-time high in the 1960's when cries of *Uhuruh* and liberation rang throughout the land. As a feminist, a sociologist, and an underpaid female professor, I was willing and eager to join the movement, but, oh God! I was appalled at the deliberate uglification of my "sisters"!

Indeed it is true that dress is a political statement. White gloves and flowered hats implied stuffy conservatism if not outright Republicanism, whereas blue jeans implied libertarianism, liberation, and liberal Democrats. But they were ugly. Granted the movement got rid of white gloves and flowered hats and girdles, and showed us how silly we were to worry about fixing up our hair and ignore what went on inside our heads. But blue jeans and tank tops were still ugly.

Many women were sympathetic to the aims of the women's liberation movement but repelled by the outward dress of its leaders. While abortion reform and day-care centers are important to many women, giving up pretty dresses was almost too high a price to pay. But once again we saw the iron hand of fashion taking over. Gloria Steinem was chic with her aviator glasses, shiny long hair, and lithe body. Blue jeans invaded Saks and Lord and Taylor's. The ultimate in reverse snobbery and reverse marketing occurred when Pierre Cardin brought out his $75 blue jeans for the young Neiman Marxists. The forty-year-old feminists who are still schlepping around Berkeley in blue jeans have lost out to slim, cool cat-packers on New York's East Side or Chicago's Golden Mile in *their* Cardin jeans or the Gucci bag packers in Bethesda.

But blue jeans are out and clinging jersey and swirling Qiana are in. Women's magazines are now playing up the new role model of glamorous lady lawyers and cool lady stockbrokers who perform their brainy tasks coiffed by Sassoon and dressed by Diane von Furstenberg. Is it once more a plot of the garment trade and Madison Avenue? Is it again a manifestation of Western bourgeois capitalism? Perhaps. But more important, fashion is fun. Women like to paint and bedeck themselves—just as women always have.

Yet we should look at all sides of the beauty culture and woman's world to analyze where the fun part of fashion may be and wherein there really lies a racket. Unsuspecting women are bilked of thousands, nay millions, of dollars a year. It is a sad comment on American culture that more money is spent in one year on cosmetics, wigs, and hair-dressers than on public education. Are American women enslaved by calorie counting and cream rinses? Why do American women willingly pay millions of dollars to diet clubs and fat farms—only to be ridiculed and humiliated? How do we absorb these rules of behavior and modes of conduct?

First of all, we are products of certain rules and traditions. Brides must wear white, unless it is the second marriage and then the "bride" must never wear white. Black is ordained for funerals, but it's ghastly taste for a wedding. Styles change—obviously, or else we would still be running around wearing bearskins and painting our bodies blue. So now women don't wear hats to church and little girls don't go off to Sunday school with white gloves. Supreme Court judges wear black robes. Professors march in processions in black robes with swaying monks' hoods denoting their school, academic discipline, and type of degree. We can well understand those kinds of rules for ceremonial occasions like weddings, funerals, Supreme Court appearances, and college graduation. What about everyday rules?

A woman who dresses "too young" is an object of ridicule. So is a professional who dresses like a Radcliffe hippie. Class, status, and a measure of power are shown in the clothes we wear or do not wear. Or our hair styles. Or our makeup. You do not wear an evening dress to the office. Long, drippy false eyelashes, red crimson lipstick, bleached hennaed hair, and a silicone bosom imply either the world's oldest profession or a stripper or some poor secretary on the make.

We are imbued with appropriate manners of speaking, dressing, acting, and painting ourselves. Our norms come to us courtesy of our mothers, grandmothers, aunts, female cousins, friends, women's fashion magazines, television commercials, movies, and window-shopping. The mass media constantly change standards of dress and makeup. therein is the consumer trap. Hemlines go up and shoulder padding goes out. Hemlines go down and necklines drop. Milady has to go out and buy a new dress. She buys a new dress and the garment industry is secure, wholesale and retail merchants are happy, and Master Charge has another 12 percent added to its coffers.

But all is not a plot and not all of us are robots. Periodically Paris or Seventh Avenue will come out with something so outrageously ugly that customers refuse to buy. Then wholesalers are unhappy and retailers go bankrupt. At least we have *some* evidence that we don't all march to the same tune of merchandise princes. But most of us agree about body size and body shape.

Fat is bad. Thin is good. And that seems to be a fairly standard Western European tradition. Overweight women have never been particularly popular, Rubens notwithstanding. Even during the Lillian Russell/Diamond Jim Brady era, a full, bosomy figure was outlined into an hourglass with a tiny wasp waist. Empress Catherine of Russia and Queen Victoria were slim-hipped, lithe, and rather sexy young women, but age and overweight ruined that image for subject, lover, and husband.

Women are constantly told and continually believe that the body beautiful guarantees upward social mobility or at least marital stability. We nod our heads in agreement with jet-setter/cat-packer Babe Paley's folk wisdom that "you can never be too rich or too thin." Body size and social class are intertwined. A woman's waistline measurement is inversely proportional to her husband's income. There are few fatties in the country club. Body size controls destiny. Blaze Starr, Lana Turner, the curvaceous chorine who married the millionaire—such are the plots of feminine Horatio Alger stories. Doors open for the shapely but close to the chubby.

Numerous studies show that fat girls with high grades are rejected by college after college, and denied admittance to the WAC and nursing schools. A few years ago there was a television show called *Arnie* about a blue-collar supervisor who had risen to middle corporate management. He was such an anomaly that he had to make do with all the leftovers. Whom did he have for a secretary? The fattest, tubbiest reject of the typing pool, of course. It really isn't too funny on or off the air for an intelligent, good, but very overweight typist never to make it even *into* the typing pool.

However, overweight and social class are highly related. Poverty food is high in starch and so poor women, especially black women, are often grossly overweight. In fact, overweight black women are consistently portrayed as the "Big Mama" with not-too-covert racial/racist overtones. Thus social class differences and racism provide some clues to understanding American insanity in regard to weight control. Fat is ugly but it is ugly because it represents social status failure, not just psychological maladjustment.

Men are not exempt from Madison Avenue gabble. Toupees, elevator shoes, wide versus narrow ties, single- versus double-breasted suits. But despite the occasional flurry over Nehru jacket, turtleneck shirt, and zippered shoes, women probably suffer more anxiety over body image and beauty than do men. We do know that there is a sociology of height for men. Men over six feet are more likely to be hired and are promoted faster than little short Napoleon types. Also police forces, military academies, and the State Department explicitly require that applicants must be free of facial scars or "any obvious deformities." We don't want Quasimodo as ambassador or general.

So Senator Proxmire and Hugh Downs get hair transplants. Men go to hair-styling salons and attend yoga classes. Part of the search for the body beautiful is the need for physical exercise in a sedentary urban environment. Proxmire jogs four miles a day to his Senate office for publicity, weight control, and as an anti-heart attack measure. While part of this book rails at America's dieting mania, we do not advocate overweight. Yet an obsession with body size and calorie and carbohydrate counting can be a sickness too.

However, most people agree that overweight is basically evil and contrary to American beauty standards. Again we point out that body size does vary from social class to social class. The mass media reflect these social class and ethnic differences. A quick glance at magazines on your local newsstand will show the difference. The most curvaceous, well-endowed women are found in photographs on the pages of detective magazines and girlie books, while the slimmest women of all are in *Vogue* and *Harper's Bazaar*. It is interesting that the women's magazines show skinnier models than men's magazines. Even the ultimate in pulchritude—the *Playboy* Playmate of the Month—is voluptuous. Not fat, but at least bosomy.

But there is one consistent item with all the models in all the magazines. Youth. They are all young. Youth madness prevails in North America. If thin is good, thin and young is better. While the Chinese apparently revere their elderly and venerate old age, Americans worship youth, lustiness, zestiness, and the sheer exuberance of the young.

It is ironic that the Haydens and Rubins who warned their peers not to trust anyone over thirty are now middle-aged themselves. And so we try to stop the aging process by whatever means are possible. Those means include hair transplants, diets, dyes, bleaches, cosmetic surgery, a new hair style to match the models in the magazines, a pair of cowboy boots, or an Ultrasuede dress. Style and fashion will halt the passage of time, and wrinkles will disappear.

However, our seeming idiocy is not news. We are the receptors of many generations of women (and men) preoccupied with personal appearance, body size, hair styles, and staving off the march of time. Fashion and body decoration are cultural imperatives. Scarification, tattoos, the Pharaoh's Afro wigs, kohl on eyelids, henna on hands and hair, farthingales, frilly garters, hoopskirts, perukes, and bustles—the list is long and esoteric for each time or generation. It is impossible to decide whether past or present generations are more masochistic.

Victorian women had their lower ribs surgically removed so that they could obtain a tiny wasp waist, while modern-day females undergo nose bobs and silicone breast implants, or have their bottoms pared off. Our great-grandmothers ate a pinch of arsenic now and then for a pale complexion, while some of today's women become addicted to the diet doctor's rainbow pills. We are subject to daily messages from television, magazines, well-meaning friends, and popular songs telling us that beauty is basic, youth is forever, and beware if you ever let up. Frank Sinatra moans a warning that an untidy housewife may lose her husband to "the girls at the office."

Preying on the housewife or working woman's fears, hopes, fantasies, and bugaboos, Madison Avenue salves their jitters. Ugly ducklings can be transformed into reasonably chic swans. How? By buying a certain face cream, joining a particular diet club, buying a particular style of blouse as advertised in *Vogue*, or flying off to a wildly expensive spa. You name it, and there is a solution—or at least most of us think so. Your life will be revamped and a new glamorous YOU will emerge from a cocoon of real or imagined ugliness.

Thus we can understand the ever-popular and recurrent articles in ladies' magazines that deal with an ugly "before" and a seductive and fashionable "after." The "before" is usually a washed-out dumpling with outdated clothes. A swift haircut by Kenneth, a new wardrobe by Bergdorf Goodman, a makeup job by Francesco, and more than likely a good night's sleep before the final photography session, and Miss Mouse of the Typing Pool becomes Ms. Junior Editorial Assistant.

The media message concerns itself not only with make-overs courtesy of certain products, but emphasizes the fact that constant vigilance combined with hard work will produce a new and lovelier you. The message is in accord with American values.

Our impossible dreams can be realized through hard work and motivation—so goes the homily on which American society is predicated. Narcissism and puritanism are linked together in an unholy and uneasy alliance, for American women are convinced that success can be achieved through beauty. Thus, if we huff, puff, starve, singe our hair, and pay enough money, we should be rewarded with radiant grace. Indeed we can mask, if not stop, the onslaught of wrinkles in the cruel light of morning. Some of us worry less, but most of us more. Weight control, deep lines, crow's-feet, and a slipping derriere are added to worries about mortgage payments and imminent invasion by the Red Chinese. Worst of all—beauty and brains are now a new goal.

It used to be written on tablets of gold that an intellectual female looked a little butchy, dressed in flat sensible shoes, wore knee socks and a suit made out of old Brillo pads. Enter the new woman! Dr. Joyce Brothers, Germaine Greer, and Gloria Steinem became darlings of the media because these women are talented *and* beautiful.

Once again, however, I ignore the sheer fun of fashion. It is exhilarating to buy a new evening gown and swish through a cocktail party. Fads, fashions, crazes, and utter silliness are the nonsensical joy of painting your face or curling your hair. My first task on moving to a new city—before checking out houses or finding a good garage mechanic—is to find the best hairdresser as soon as possible. If you look good, you feel good. Or at least that's the way I feel. It's my hair and my neurosis. But I'm not alone. Women in the Western world in the 1970's are concerned over the burning issues of dress and hair style. So what does it all mean?

We have standards of beauty for Grecian urns and film festivals and so why not for people? If a woman (or man) follows the *media via*, a little bit of narcissism is healthy. If Narcissus had only peeked in the pool, his untimely demise would have been delayed. It's when women unwittingly swallow advertising's gibberish and devote every waking moment to attaining unattainable standards that they are mutilated in both body and soul.

The radical critique of fashion says that adherence to

beauty standards is a manifestation of bourgeois mentality. But when everyone runs around in shapeless baggy blue Mao jackets and floppy baggy pants, it *is* awfully boring. The Chinese have recently introduced fashion shows and several acceptable dresses for the people of the People's Republic. It blew New Left radical North American women's minds when they visited Cuba and found that the Cuban women's militia trained with machine guns by day and took lessons in hair style and makeup by night. American lefties—in boots, jeans, and jean jackets, with long stringy hair—couldn't comprehend what makeup and hair styles meant to the Cuban militia women. It really is very simple.

Before the revolution, working women or at least sugarcane- and factory-working women had little time or inclination to learn the latest fashion modes. Only the middle- and upper-class bourgeoisie women could indulge themselves. So cometh the revolution and olive-drab-clad revolutionary women wield sugarcane knives, machine guns, and eyebrow pencils.

So also do women in the American armed services. I have been on field training exercises with WAC officers and enlisted women in the U.S. Army and seen army women touching up their lipstick in freezing weather. While army fatigues are hardly the epitome of high fashion, a little lipstick or a smudge of olive-drab eyeshadow helps to relieve monotony and raise morale of male and female soldier alike.

No one tells army women that they should wear makeup, only that it must be "in good taste." Most do wear makeup. Some WACs in the field make elaborate and heartbreaking efforts to curl or set their hair. Why not? They are soldiers and women. The two are not antithetical. These are young women who have learned that makeup and hair styles are "proper," "right," or "the appropriate way of behaving and acting." Curly hair and a smidge of makeup mean that you are a well-turned-out young person.

This helps explain why the first signs of depression in a woman are whenever a woman neglects her personal appearance. Stringy, unwashed hair, baggy stockings with runs in them, unkempt clothing, no makeup—these are outward signs of inward turmoil. But beware when the terribly depressed woman suddenly fixes herself up. She goes to the hairdresser, buys a new dress, cleans the house thoroughly, puts on her new dress, and calmly kills herself.

Women's sense of self is so wrapped up in the body-image syndrome that female suicides rarely disfigure themselves. That's why women more often use pills to commit suicide and not the preferred male suicide weapon—a gun. The female suicide is most likely to get fully clothed (in that new dress) and lie peacefully on the bed awaiting whatever fate the pills bring her.

Because of this recurring pattern of behavior, therapists have long been sensitive to cues of a woman's hair, dress, makeup, or general overall appearance. Most mental hospitals have a beauty parlor tucked away somewhere in the building. Psychiatrists and psychologists know that when a woman looks horrible, she often feels and acts horrible. And when facilities are not available to help a woman look better, she often sinks into a deeper and deeper depression.

So beauty parlors in psychiatric hospitals and prisons cater not to the whims of fashion but to cultural imperatives of woman's culture. Women are socialized differently from men, so their therapeutic or rehabilitative process has to take into account those important aspects of a woman's life—her self-image as projected by dress and demeanor.

Several years ago I listened to the warden of a large federal women's prison expound on how she had brought New York models, hair stylists, cosmetologists, fashion consultants, and speech coaches to her prison. She said that she wanted her prisoners to learn how to dress, speak, walk, and act like nice middle-class girls. The general impression the audience received was that, if you could give a swinging floosie lessons on dress and deportment, her chances for a middle-class job would be increased. Sort of an Eliza Doolittle syndrome in federal prison. But the lady warden was much more realistic than her starry-eyed social worker audience.

The lady warden explained her plan in a nutshell. ''Enter hooker, exit call girl,'' she said. Then the warden explained further. She pointed out that prostitution was the most viable occupation for these women, since they had no education, training, skills, or marketable talents. These girls were never in prison long enough to make up their schooling or learn a trade. Besides, prostitution paid well and was not subject to income tax. However, there is a hierarchy of values, salaries, rewards and punishments between streetwalkers and call girls. The warden pointed out that call girls have less alcoholism, less drug addiction, less venereal disease, and a much lower suicide rate than streetwalkers. So the warden decided if she were going to improve the life-style of her inmates, she would teach them to be polite, demure, well-dressed, and fashionably attired middle-class ladies. Thus the phrase, ''Enter hooker, exit call girl.''

Even though the therapeutic community was attuned to woman's world and woman's culture, it still was not a subject that social scientists wanted to discover. The exotica of an Arabian harem was titillating but the inner sanctum of an upper-upper-class beauty salon was not. Dissertations abound on the masochistic meaning of medieval monks flagellating themselves. No one ever bothered to dissect the psychological meaning of machines that torture and pound people every day in chains of spas and exercise salons. Researchers combed Appalachia for ballads and poems, while only a few people paid any attention to soap operas or women's magazines.

Those few social scientists or English professors who delved into the normal everyday life of most women usually loved to point with glee at the idiocy of soap-opera plot or the stupidity of a predominantly female audience.

Since I was part of woman's culture and also a member of the social science community, I persisted in trying to sort out the meanings of this woman's world. How do we learn the ''right'' ways of dressing? What does it mean to be a woman in the 1970's? How different are we today from ladies of Louis XIV's court? How proscribed and pre-scribed are we in our actions?

With these questions in mind, I turned to a detailed analysis of some parts of woman's culture. At the same time the reader should remember that I am part of this same culture and bound by the same rules and proscriptions as anyone else. Even though I am a social scientist and supposed to remain aloof from my subject, it is hard to be dispassionate when uncovering fraud.

Some, if not most, of the merchants in this woman's world deliberately lie, defraud, mislead, and con their clientele. Patent medicine and medical quacks promise a quick cure to Ms. America's obesity. Magic wafers, diet candy, kelp pills, wheat germ, and Vitamin B are touted as diet aids. Even though the AMA intones its warnings and the FDA charges some drug companies, the diet doctors thrive. They flourish because, as in other dishonest activities—gambling, confidence rackets, or selling of narcotics—the victims demand that they continue. Diet doctors, whether of the medical or osteopathic or chiropractic variety, persist because desperate women come to them begging for relief from fat. Women get their amphetamines, digitalis, thyroid, and harsh diuretics along with blinding headaches, personality changes, nausea, vomiting, fainting spells, and tingling of the hands and feet. Sometimes they even lose weight too.

American women spend hours counting calories, cook their brains out under hair dryers, search for the perfect little black dress, chatter endlessly about the current diet fad, and rage at their slowly aging and always imperfect reflection. Why not? Such behavior is perfectly understandable given a society that bombards its women with messages that they must be beautiful in order to "succeed."

Feminists usually deride beauty standards and demand that women cast aside Madison Avenue and refuse to follow fashion. Yet my feminist sisters were also not quite honest in their supposed rejection of fashion and style. I began to notice that blue jeans and loose flowing hair might be the uniform for the day but nighttime was another matter. My radical feminist sisters changed their demeanor and style of dress from afternoon to evening. The nighttime feminist was dressed in long skirt, piled her hair high on her head, bedecked herself with jewelry, and wore tasteful makeup.

This new woman may be the salvation of our egos. If you are happy and comfortable in your clothes and like yourself or your hair style, as the Jews say—Mazeltov! When fashion is fun, when a new color of lipstick makes you feel better, when a new hair color boosts your ego, then fashion is good. Often when tension mounts in my office and tempers run rampant, I spend my lunch hour in the beauty salon. I remove myself from office tension, become soothed, petted, and pampered, and return to the office calmer and really quite happier.

My trip to the hairdresser is cheaper therapy than going to a shrink. However, as we shall see later, psychotherapists and hair stylists often perform the same function. As I began to analyze my own motives for sneaking off to the hairdresser or wondered why I felt guilty about watching soap operas, my curiosity led me even further into woman's world.

This is a culture that stretches across age, sex, racial, and social class barriers. We learn from early childhood what clothes or makeup are appropriate for a particular age or social class group. As a matter of fact we are really indoctrinated at birth with a pink blanket and a pink baby identification bracelet. Little boys really shouldn't have long curls past age three but little girls should. Little girls are supposed to be cleaner and neater than little boys—and mothers usually make sure that's what happens. Little girls play for hours with mother's makeup and dress up in high heels and mother's gloves and dresses. Whenever a little boy tries to emulate his mother or older sister by putting on lipstick or dressing up in mother's clothes, his horrified relatives put a screeching halt to his play.

Little boys learn quickly and forcefully that girls paint their fingernails and lips, boys do not. Girls put curlers in their hair, boys do not. Probably the parents' reactions the first time a boy tries to put on lipstick are so violent that a boy learns that there is something shameful about putting on lipstick. The shameful part is of course that the parents are worried sick about their son's becoming a homosexual. So both boys and girls learn that painting your face and dressing up in mommy's clothes are good things for girls and bad things for boys.

Girls learn that "dressing up" *is* a lot of fun. A little girl prancing before her mother's dresser in mommy's dress grows up to be an excited young woman who twirls before the department store mirror in her bridal gown. Dress marks every important milestone in our lives. Christening robes, Girl Scout uniforms, prom dresses, wedding gowns, cocktail dresses, mother-of-the-bride dresses, and whatever someone chooses for the final laying-out ceremony. Of course you can have a closet full of clothes and still frantically wail to your husband, ''I have nothing to wear.''

It may be that the styles have changed so radically that you really don't have anything to wear. Or at least nothing that is in accord with current modes. Maybe you are a recent college graduate and really don't have anything to wear because you have never been invited to a formal tea before. There are some really good reasons why you can say that you have nothing to wear.

Or you may be like me and need some sort of excuse to wander around the boutiques and buy something new. Buying and shopping are therapeutic to most women. Mothers indoctrinate their girl children into the shopping syndrome by taking the little girls along on expeditions to the department stores. Little boys don't get taken along because they don't behave as well, are more restless, and usually raise a fuss. That doesn't mean that little girls don't get equally as restless but they are forced to behave better. Little girls behave better because mothers don't tolerate the same kind of nonsense from a girl as from a boy. Little girls soon learn that firm retribution comes to a restless, badly behaved child. The little boy learns if he misbehaves he gets left at home. And that's where he wants to be anyway.

So mommy and daughter make forays into the shopping malls. Some psychologists say that shopping is the feminine equivalent of voyeurism for men. Who knows? But we do know that women do like to shop much more than men do. Daughters learn about style of dress or hair through their long trips with their mothers. Little girls see their mothers poring over books and magazines. Then the little girl begins to absorb messages from television regarding what is a good-looking person.

Black leaders were quite aware how insidious these mass-media messages could be—and were—and are. Television commercials, advertisements in books and magazines, models on billboard posters, photographs in sales brochures, actors on soap operas and evening drama shows were nearly exclusively white fifteen years ago. Today, in spite of a concerted campaign to include black models and actors in advertising and television, the number of blacks still remains small. Even though black pride coined the phrase "Black is beautiful," WASPy standards of beauty prevail.

Movies, television, magazine and book illustrations tell us that only good-looking people buy Cadillacs, smoke Kents, drink Coca-Cola, and sip Grants. Most of these good-looking people are slim-hipped Caucasians—and usually blond. So if you are a Jewish girl with a big nose, a swarthy-skinned Italian girl, a black woman with a frizzy Afro, or an overweight WASP, you sure are out of the running. Or are you?

No, you are not. Because Madison Avenue shows you how to get the ideal body type and hair color. And now we have our entrée to the strange and exotic woman's culture of the United States.

2 Carbohydrate Counters

It is a sin to be fat in the United States. Not only is corpulence unsightly and an affront to morale, but it is a sign of sloth, self-indulgence, and lack of discipline. At least that's what mass advertising, your friends, and diet-club lecturers tell you.

Nearly 79 million people in the United States are overweight. Five thousand doctors devote themselves exclusively to weight control. Nearly $400 million is spent on reducing drugs. If we include the money spent on reducing aids, diet books, diet clubs, diet magazines, and exercise aids, the figure jumps to over a billion dollars a year! Dieting is a national obsession in the United States and has developed into the second-favorite indoor sport.

With nearly one-third of the population of the United States dieting, going on a diet, thinking about dieting, or recovering from dieting depression, journalists, medical doctors, physiologists, and the average-man-on-the-street all expound with equal fervor their pet theories on obesity. People are fat because:

- they have malfunctioning glands.
- they have a preponderance of "fat cells."
- they don't exercise enough.
- fat runs in their family.
- everything they eat turns to fat.
- they eat too much.
- they eat too many sweets and carbohydrates.
- they eat when they get nervous.

The clue, of course, is that obesity results from calories ingested in relation to calories expended. Ergo: Lumberjacks eat mammoth amounts of food but stay relatively trim. A housewife, however, who eats like a lumberjack is a heart-attack candidate, probably a Lane Bryant customer, and most likely miserably unhappy.

And the more food she eats, the bigger she gets and the more she hates herself. The United States is a thin society. Ms. Average is constantly reminded on TV, in magazines, in store windows, and on the street that thin women are beautiful women. Fat women are ugly. Pills, belts, reducing machines, wafers, diet candy, diet soda, saccharin, sauna baths, and calorie charts scream out the message that excess flesh is repugnant. The woman hates herself, is sure that other people hate her, and hides at home ashamed of her body. But at the same time, she is convinced that she is pretty and that she would be gorgeous if only she weren't so fat.

When she finally decides to diet, the overweight woman rushes to the bookstore for the current fad diet book, to the dime store for a calorie counter or a carbohydrate wheel, to the drugstore for appetite depressants, and she is on her way. Why not? She is a professional dieter. Nearly every carbohydrate counter (or CC'er for short) has followed one of the many fad diets to come to the fore in the past few years. Rice diet; grapefruit and egg diet; soybean and evaporated milk diet; coffee, grapefruit, and yoga: All are successful. The crazier the diet, the more successful it seems. Often, as with the Doctor's Quick Weight Loss Diet, many television appearances by the author, in this case Dr. Stillman, give credibility to the diet. All these diets work because they involve no magic "burning up of calories," just reduction in calories. The CC'er is a professional dieter who usually skips breakfast and lunch in order to lose weight. She can go on protracted fasts for several days and lose weight with ease. But starving or drinking Stillman's ten glasses of water or choking down the greasy evaporated milk laced with soybean oil becomes tedious if not downright impossible. She watches her calories, counts her carbohydrates, gags on her umpteenth hard-boiled egg, and weighs herself constantly.

Even though it has taken years for her to pile on her thirty, fifty, or one hundred extra pounds, she wants to lose five pounds between 8:00 A.M. and 2:00 P.M. When the scales fail to register a loss for one or two days, she finally says, "To hell with it," and goes on a binge to end all binges. Ice cream, beer, pizza, Polish sausage, and angel food cake: You name it and she'll eat it. She'll not eat it, she'll *devour* it. (When movie star Judy Holliday dieted she cleared out all food from her house, but when she got the urge for a binge she would eat dog food in order to satisfy her craving.) An obese person on a binge is a woman possessed of a thousand devils. She races through the kitchen opening and closing cupboard doors searching for food. She eats with both hands; she stuffs food into her mouth until she looks like a squirrel storing nuts for the winter; and she hates herself every minute for what she is doing.

Berating herself, crying for shame, vomiting for self-punishment, and promising herself never to repeat her past errors, a chastened fattie asks if there is not a better way to lose weight. She reads one more ad in a newspaper, or hears one more promise on the radio, and decides to take one more chance. She'll join Carbohydrate Counters.

Carbohydrate Counters is a not-so-mythical organization whose description is based on research into nationally franchised weight-reducing clubs such as Weight Watchers, TOPS (Take Off Pounds Sensibly), Overeaters Anonymous, etc., and many private local diet clubs.[1] Diet clubs perform the same function for the food addict as Alcoholics Anonymous and Synanon do for their members. Group therapy, group support, public confession, a reformed, rehabilitated leader, a strict regimen, and sympathy for the backslider form the base of CC structure. To join CC, the prospective member must be at least twenty pounds overweight, agree to attend weekly meetings, and follow the diet faithfully.

The examination of our thinly disguised organization is based on two years of observations and results of a series of questionnaires distributed to a local diet club. How does the diet club work? What needs does it fulfill for the members—other than providing diet rules? Is it a unique female society in and of itself?

Although most members come to Carbohydrate Counters as a last-ditch, going-down-for-the-third-time last resort, they are still not convinced that they can adjust to dieting. Often members admit that they went on food binges the week before joining so that they could have their last fling with food. Some members come to their first meeting drunk because they cannot face the shame of weighing in before a stranger who will not accept the rationalizations and excuses that their families have swallowed for too many years.

> Before I decided to join CC I went to a family reunion and ate everything that was out at the picnic. There were long tables that went the length and breadth of the buffet and I kept going up and down them and piling up my plate. I ate and ate. Then I went back and ate some more. I knew that I would never be able to adjust to the CC diet without having had the memory of one last orgy of food.
>
> (thirty-eight-year-old female)

Class size fluctuates according to the season of the year. Classes are decimated in November and December because members refuse to come in during periods of ritually ordained feasting. In January, membership dramatically increases in direct proportion to New Year's resolutions about losing weight. When the obese face the grisly thought of another summer at the beach with a beach towel covering up the size 16 bathing suit, classes increase in April and May. Summer is low point for membership because the majority of the members have to face their cover-up summer on the beach and won't diet if they can't wear a bikini *now.* Fall sees an upsurge in membership because the overweights dream about fitting into a slinky sequined dress for New Year's Eve. And so it goes on and on.

The ups and downs of membership rolls parallel the yo-yo syndrome of patron's gains and losses. If the dieter adheres to the game plan, weight losses result. (But if *any* diet or reduction in calories occurs, poundage disappears.) What is the secret of a diet club such as the Carbohydrate Counters? How is CC able to succeed with dieters who have a long history of failure?

Carbohydrate Counters is patterned on the research of Norman Jolliffe, M.D., who developed his "Prudent Diet" while director of the New York City Bureau of Nutrition, Department of Health.[2] Recognizing that there is only a minute number of persons with severe glandular disorders, Dr. Jolliffe realized that the compulsive eaters were often ignorant of basic nutrition and needed complete retraining of their eating habits. To retrain anyone for anything is miracle enough, and for the overweight, well-nigh impossible. But Jolliffe did it.

Jolliffe's diet includes foods from those "basic groups" that we all learned about in seventh grade home economics, Girl Scouts, or boring health classes. Green leafy vegetables, red and yellow vegetables, proteins, fruits, carbohydrates, milk, and enriched bread—there is nothing new in that. Jolliffe's fillips involved a heavy concentration of fish, low fat, and some interesting recipes. The basic pattern in Jolliffe's diet that was transformed into CC dogma and liturgy is five fish, three beef, and one liver meal a week. Women should have three fruits daily, men five, and one of them must be citrus.

Again, there is no surprise in these dietary admonitions.

Jolliffe coined the word "appestat" (a combination of appetite and thermostat) to denote the appetite-regulating mechanism located in the hypothalamus gland. Normal people eat until they are satisfied or "filled." The obese eat and eat and eat. Their appestat either doesn't function or is giving misdirected cues telling the body that it has to continue eating. Given that many overweight people overeat for psychological reasons, dieting is a trauma. Taking food away from the compulsive eater produces the same reaction as taking heroin away from the addict.

Jolliffe achieved weight losses in his patients by transmogrifying the neurotic eater into the neurotic dieter. Prior to beginning the Jolliffe diet, the overweight person stuffed herself with chocolate or greasy pork; after the Jolliffe regimen, she stuffed herself with asparagus or lettuce. The Prudent Diet is strict, authoritarian, and nondeviating. Dieters are given certain free foods such as bouillon or unflavored gelatin. They may eat huge quantities of low-calorie vegetables such as asparagus, pimentos, spinach, watercress, and radishes. Carbohydrate Counters spend endless hours figuring out their shopping lists, weighing their food on especially purchased postage scales, poring over recipe books, talking on the telephone to fellow CC'ers, and attending weekly meetings.

The weekly meetings are the core secret of CC's victory in the battle of the bulge. Members pay an initiation fee of about five dollars and a weekly fee usually of three dollars. Any member who misses a week must pay for the missed week or weeks. While CC is a money-making organization itself, small local imitators have found that charging fees is a necessity, even if the meetings are held in private homes, because the American money-oriented public seems to have little time for an organization that doesn't charge. Members will skip coming to meetings when they have cheated, and CC leaders feel sure that if no fee were charged for missed meetings more backsliding would occur. Members line up to pay their weekly fee and then stand in line waiting to be weighed.

What first strikes the new member on entering the CC meeting is the noise level. CC meetings are noisy with members chattering, giggling, and nervously hee-hawing at each other's pathetic jokes. People that are food-oriented (or orally fixated, according to Freudians) like to talk a great deal. Members babble on endlessly about their dieting success or their inability to control their penchant for double-layer fudge nut torte. But CC language is a peculiar argot confusing to the neophyte. CC'ers do not "diet," they "stay on program." When they have not cheated on program, they are said to be "legal." And when they reach their desired weight, they have "attained goal." Burbling over their legal foods or free foods, their newest recipes, they wait for their moment of redemption or retribution—the scales.

Each member tries to dress in her lightest clothing so as not to affect the scales. The majority of CC'ers are forty-year-old women; a handful of teen-agers, young married women, men, and pensioners are scattered here and there. Dressed in their housedresses, too-tight jeans, or snug suits, these people exhibit some common traits. CC meetings are the last outpost of the bouffant hairdo combed into bouncy curls on top of the head that bobs in rhythm with the member's jouncing bosom. Leaving a trail of bobby pins as they move up in line, CC'ers from the rear look as though their derrieres are large paper bags with two small boys inside fighting to get out. Plucking at their rhinestone pins, fiddling with their rhinestone earrings, clutching at their overblouses, straightening their peekaboo bra straps, and biting their nails, they chew gum more and more furiously while their smiles turn to grimaces as they prepare for the scales.

Weighing in is the moment of truth, a trauma. It's when the bullfighter meets the bull, or more aptly, when the heifer steps on the scale. Without exception, each member comes to the scales, looks at the lecturer, looks at the scales, and then, in a type of genuflection, bends down before the omniscient scale and takes off her shoes. Most members begin an elaborate striptease. They remove coats, jackets, and sweaters, and leave purses on the floor. I have also seen members take off their earrings and girdles. One woman, in a gesture of sheer desperation, snatched off her wig when the scales didn't measure a loss. Part of the weighing-in ritual is to argue with the scale clerk over the relative merits of the member's bathroom scale versus the large, imposing "doctor's scale" used by the CC club. Some lecturers get so furious over the repeated imprecations about, "Well my scale at home says that I'm three pounds lighter than this scale. There has to be something wrong with this scale," that they tell members not to weigh at home. One lecturer says that she advises all members to wrap up their scale in newspaper, put it in a box, wrap the box up with brown paper, string, and gobs of brown paper tape, put the box under the bed, and then forget that there is a scale in the house. She says that by the time the member has wrapped, unwrapped, and rewrapped the scale several times, she will be content to weigh herself only at CC meetings once a week.

But that member is rare. Even among the lecturers, weighing only once a week is rare. Stepping on the scales and recording weight is a continual procedure. I have seen lecturers weigh themselves five times in a one-hour period. The same lecturers who admonish their members regarding weighing at home seem to go berserk when in the same room as a calibrated scale. Lecturers and members alike anthropomorphize the scale as "it" or "he."

He is terrible. He tells the truth. That thing is over there in the corner and he is looking at me. He knows if I have cheated or not. Oh, I can get him to fudge a little by shifting my weight or letting out my breath. But he usually wins.

(twenty-eight-year-old CC lecturer)

Scales are well chosen as the symbol of justice, for they do weigh and find some waning and others waxing. The lecturer can almost spot cheaters, because they come to the weighing-in ceremony with big sheepish grins on their faces and usually announce, "I was good all week." When a member tells you how "good" she has been, that's usually an indication that she's been bad. One young girl who admitted that she had "cheated a little," burst into tears when the scales announced a five-pound gain over the past week.

It wasn't that bad. I really didn't think I done that bad. I don't know what to do. It was only a little chicken.

When asked by the lecturer how little was a "little chicken," the girl retorted angrily, "I told you, a *little* chicken." The lecturer insisted on knowing how much was a little chicken: "Show me with your hands what a little chicken is." The sixteen-year-old held out her arms at right angles to her body and said, "Here, damn it. This is a little chicken." Little for a turkey maybe, but a big, big chicken.

Leaving the scale room, each member is quizzed by her friends as to whether she gained or lost. Those who lost announce their losses, even if it was half a pound or a quarter of a pound. A common CC joke is that a quarter of a pound equals one stick of butter. Those who have not lost will mutter about legal gains or menstrual period only to be reminded by a friend that this is the third week in a row that she has had a menstrual period. Some of the excuses are ingenious:

"I had an automobile accident four days ago, and you wouldn't believe how upset I have been. I've just been frantic and I certainly didn't stick with program."

"We went camping and you can't be legal in a trailer far from the store."

But most are simply mundane run-of-the-mill apologies:

"I have gland problems."

"I come from a family of big people."

"I'm big-boned."

Apparently, fat persons are unable to refuse food on special occasions such as their own birthday, a graduation, wedding, or when the buzzards come back to Hinkle, Iowa.

What is interesting is that often the wife will tell the weigh-in clerk how her husband urges her to eat fattening foods. One weigh-in clerk finally snapped at one such woman, "What you ought to do is get rid of that bastard and then you could lose weight." The next week, the patron came in, weighed in, and had lost five pounds. Congratulated by the weigh-in clerk, the member smirked and said, "I really lost one hundred and eighty-five pounds." The clerk was somewhat confused and asked, "What do you mean?" "Well, I took your advice. I got rid of the bastard.

I figured that he was deliberately trying to keep me fat so that he could have a good time needling me about my lack of willpower. It took me twenty years to figure it out but I'm well rid of him."

While some women have nasty husbands, many have equally vicious friends. One evening as I was weighing Mrs. Smith, she burst into tears because, although she had been legal all week long and had expected to register a loss on the scales, instead she had a ten-pound gain. I was as disturbed as Mrs. Smith until I noticed that Mrs. Smith's "friend," Mrs. Robinson, was standing with *her* foot on the scale. Mrs. Smith treated the incident with remarkable calm, since she was so relieved to find out that she had actually lost weight and not gained. The two women began to kid each other and poke each other in the ribs. The reason for Mrs. Robinson's behavior was apparent when she stepped on the scale and showed a three-pound gain. Mrs. Robinson didn't want her legal friend, Mrs. Smith, to enjoy her triumph without a moment of panic.

If competition between two friends who are dieting strains the bonds of friendship, think what happens to the mother-daughter relationship. Fashion-conscious mothers often drag their unwilling and overweight daughters to CC meetings ostensibly for the benefit of the daughter. The mother is usually a professional dieter who gains and loses weight at will, while the daughter is most often a pudgy, timid lump living in her overpowering mother's reflection. The mother sees the worst of her own personality and body reproduced in the daughter. The mother doesn't really want the daughter to lose weight because then there will be a svelte rival in the home. As long as the daughter remains fat, the mother's position as sex goddess is secure. The mother uses her diet as a weapon to prove continually to the daughter that momma is made of much sterner stuff than her weak-willed daughter, whom the mother berates for being "just like your father."

It is pathetically simple. If the CC member sticks to the diet (or if anyone sticks to any diet), she will lose weight. For CC'ers, their diet—or program—is endowed with mystical qualities. No deviations are allowed because there is supposedly a "chemical reaction" that takes place. Fad diets are despised by CC'ers, yet the CC diet (which is the Jolliffe Prudent Diet) has been elevated to the status of a cult. A strange perversion takes place between Jolliffe's books and CC lecturers' claptrap regarding the diet.

Jolliffe didn't feel that any food was absolutely necessary to the Prudent Diet, but liver and fish are now mainstays of the CC program. Liver is the bugaboo of most dieters.

> I can't eat liver. I hate it. I don't know what to do. The only way I can eat liver is smothered in fried onions and fried in butter. So I grind up the liver in the blender and drink the whole mess down in one gulp.
>
> (thirty-five-year-old female)

CC members are reluctant to eat fish. While the United States is hardly a land-locked continent, fish is not a staple in our diet. For this reason, the CC diet is often the first time many people have eaten fish on a regular basis.

For me the CC diet is a tuna fish diet. I eat tuna fish five times a week. There is no other fish that I like.

(fifty-five-year-old female)

I lost all kinds of weight on the CC diet because I ate fish all the time. I had fish maybe fifteen times a week. I had fish for breakfast, lunch, and dinner. It's the fish that makes you lose weight.

(thirty-six-year-old female)

Jolliffe knew that the more leeway a dieter is given to pick and choose his foods, the more cheating will take place. But if someone wants to lose weight, she can do so by holding herself to 1,000 to 1,500 calories per day, and these calories can be from ice cream, beer, peanuts, or whatever else the dieter wants to eat as long as he or she stays within the 1,000- to 1,500-calorie range. The trouble is, it's difficult to calculate the calorie count of just one little drink or just one little handful of peanuts, and sooner than you can count to 1,000, the limit has been surpassed. Jolliffe was in favor of a rigid diet giving the dieter choice only among green leafy vegetables. CC'ers follow Jolliffe's prescriptions. Some of the compulsive eaters go hog wild on the "free foods." One woman ate twelve heads of lettuce in one afternoon, another ate twenty boxes of broccoli in an evening, and many dieters report that they buy low-calorie soft drinks by the case, drinking fifteen or more daily. Nevertheless, maybe twelve heads of lettuce cause less harm than ten pounds of chocolate. Keep in mind that the compulsive eater has to be munching on something most of the time.

The compulsive eater likes to eat and likes to think about food. On the Jolliffe diet, the compulsive eater concentrates the major portion of his time and effort on buying and preparing the correct food. Low-calorie cookbooks abound. CC members bring recipes to meetings; recipes are Xeroxed and handed out; and members call the lecturers to taste their newest concoction. Truly the neurotic eater now is the neurotic dieter.

Before CC, the individual member hid food and lied about her eating habits; after joining CC, she can use her diet as an expression of hostility. Given encouragement to say "no" to her hostess or relatives, she begins to assert herself aggressively. She becomes a fanatical dieter. Rather than saying, "No, thank you," she snarls, "I can't have that! You know I can't have that! You are trying to make me go off my diet." She (or he) carries around a "survival kit" consisting of sugar substitute, salad herbs in a shaker jar, consommé packets, or homemade salad dressings. Some fanatics even carry their postal scale with them to weigh food in restaurants or private homes. Those who travel the cocktail-party circuit carry their own low-calorie soft drinks with them which enable them to withstand temptation. CC'ers who decide that they need a "fish day" will take frozen fish dinners, which they heat and self-righteously eat, when invited to a friend's home for dinner. Rather than express their hostility through stuffing themselves with forbidden high-calorie food, they lash out at the world through their dieting.

Carbohydrate Counters, like the Catholic Church, also recognizes sins of omission. Members recite a psalmody of not having enough fish meals, not eating liver, forgetting their piece of bread at noon, or skipping meals.

The sacred ceremony of public confession is one essential dynamic of CC liturgy. Members who have been ashamed of turning their lengthwise mirror sideways or too embarrassed to explain to their husbands exactly what the chocolate éclairs are doing in the clothes hamper now have an opportunity to air their opinions, fears, and secret horrors freely. No story is too wretched to be told because usually the lecturer or another member will try to top it. After having suffered from parental sarcasm, endured insensitive doctors and years of smirks from husband and children, at last the fat woman has found a haven. For the first time in years, she will take off her coat in public. Most fat people are convinced that if they keep their coats on they will look smaller, or at least people may think that the coat and not the bulky body is taking up so much space. They eagerly join in the discussion and learn that others too hide, sneak, or steal food, go on binges that they bitterly regret, dream of food, constantly weigh themselves, and loathe themselves for being fat. At one meeting of over one hundred CC members, the lecturer broke the meeting into small discussion groups and asked the members to discuss how they felt being fat. Some of their comments follow:

> We felt hot, sweaty, knew we looked terrible in clothes, felt out of control.

We agreed that fat people are slobs.

Our group all agreed that we hated ourselves for being fat but we realized how self-destructive this hate could be. Because we hated ourselves for being fat, we were unhappy, and when fat people are unhappy, they eat.

The hour grows late, the discussion more revealing, and the room hotter and hotter. Bodies begin to sweat and the smell of drugstore perfume cloys. Nerve endings are rubbed raw. The atmosphere is reminiscent of a Pentacostal revival meeting, combined with a basketball pep rally and overtones of a voodoo *houngan.* The lecturer guides and controls her class. The lecturer is CC to each member. The success or failure of each class, each area, and each franchise rests ultimately with the lecturer. The lecturer is mother, father, priest, minister, psychiatrist, nu ritionist, marriage counselor, job consultant, fashion coordinator, and comedienne all wrapped up in one tidy CC package. The lecturer is a symbol and a role model.

Who is she? What training does she have? Does she realize what power she has over the lives of so many people? Is she a help or a menace?

Lecturers who have lost fifty, a hundred, or even two hundred pounds are walking testimonials to better health, happier marriages, and the delights of following the dictates of fashion. Lecturers are on a permanent and continual ego trip with their adoring sycophantic audiences. Lecturers pirouette in front of their classes and proclaim, "Look at me. I'm beautiful. I used to be ugly but now I'm gorgeous.

If you do what I tell you to do, you can be equally as lovely and have all the advantages that I have.'' And the members are anxious to believe. CC lecturers overcome the members' reluctance to diet because, like the reformed alcoholic, the CC lecturer is a reformed foodaholic. She is similar to the Alcoholics Anonymous group leader who announces that he is a drunk, for the CC lecturer always begins her lecture by saying, ''Hi. My name is Margaret and I lost thirty-five pounds with CC.'' This opening is meant to reassure the new members that the sleek fashion plate on the dais is not a snippy little know-nothing but a reformed compulsive eater. Her example gives courage to dieters who have never been able to stick to a diet for longer than two or three weeks.

The mantle of greatness falls upon the prospective CC lecturer shortly before she is about to reach goal weight. Usually she has been a steady and noncheating member, faithfully attending classes, always well-groomed, usually witty, and unabashedly devoted to her lecturer. Lecturers enjoy reporting that they were *chosen* to be lecturers and thus CC representatives. Not one lecturer ever said that she had deliberately sought this position but rather that ''Louise had to coax me,'' or ''Esther had to beg me and persuade me to be a lecturer.'' CC lecturers revel in the fact that each was chosen for her own unique qualities.

But lecturers fit a decided pattern. A typical lecturer is a white, married female, age thirty-eight, with high school education or better, who has worked at a white-collar job, usually before her marriage, and has two children. Compared to the typical CC member, the lecturer is younger, better-educated, and has worked longer at a higher-level job.

The absolute epitome of successful dieter, ex-fattie darling of fat-club lecturers, and success of female successes is Jean Nidetch (née Slutsky) from the Bronx. Founder of Weight Watchers (or WW as the aficionados call it), Jean Nidetch weighed in at 214 pounds. Attending Norman Jolliffe's obesity clinic, Jean Nidetch took the diet and by combining her personality with strict Alcoholics Anonymous meeting procedure, she parlayed herself into a personal fortune worth approximately $6 million. There are now nine million WW'ers throughout the world. Not bad! Jean Slutsky Nidetch is Cinderella to the fat housewife. She personifies all the dreams-come-true of Mrs. Average. Wearing expensive couturier clothes, yakking it up on the talk shows, rubbing elbows with celebrities, packing audiences in with greater success than Billy Graham, metamorphosed from a dowdy nonentity faintly resembling a mattress tied in the middle, Jean Slutsky Nidetch has made it big. Jean's message is, "I did it and so can you." Franchisers and lecturers carry on in the tradition of their proselytizing prophet, for each one of them has also emerged from her respective chrysalis of fat into a well-groomed butterfly.

Diet clubs take their ex-fatties, train them, and make them into carbon copies of Jean Nidetch. These dedicated women then, in turn, recite their thanks to the diet club. Provide an example of an ex-fattie now glamour girl and the cash register clanks on and on.

CC training varies throughout the country. Some CC

lecturers attend regular Saturday morning training sessions, work as tally clerks, or scale assistants, or lecturers-in-training. Some CC area franchise owners send their lecturers to charm school to make them serve a six months' apprenticeship. Others simply give the lecturer a handshake and tell her that she starts next week. Most lecturers do have two or three all-day training sessions. Managers give lecturers a thick handbook telling CC dos and don'ts which are underscored again and again in training sessions.

Lecturers are taught how to talk, walk, sit, speak in public, and dress. Managers stress that lecturers represent CC to the public at large. As such, lecturers are expected to be well-groomed at all times, including trips to the grocery store. One lecturer-trainer admonished her trainees:

> You just can't schlep around in any old thing anymore. You are CC lecturers. In your old fat days you could go to the grocery store in your husband's jeans and his old shirt hanging out and your hair up in rollers. You are somebody. What would you do if you were trying to lose weight and you saw me wandering around, dressed in horrible dirty old clothes? You would not only think less of me, you would think that CC was really a crummy organization to let such terrible people work for it. Now, wouldn't you?

The trainees nodded their heads in agreement. Each was particularly pleased that now she was "somebody" and had many people looking up to her for encouragement and guidance. No blue jeans. Men must always wear ties. No jangling jewelry. No flashy clothes. How wonderful to be a fashion plate! CC lecturers enjoy their Cinderella metamorphosis because for many this is the first job in many years and one of the rare occasions in which their dreams have come to fruition.

Lecturers are told that they must have their "fat picture" displayed prominently so that members can see the before and after evidence of effective dieting. CC lecturers are told that they always have to tell members how many pounds they have lost. The fat picture and the "fat story" reinforce CC's effectiveness. However, the strong bonds between class and lecturer increase with every sign that the lecturer cares. It is a strong symbiotic relationship. For every ounce a member loses, she gives adulation to the lecturer who made this great moment possible.

Some lecturers take their role as missionaries so seriously that they proselytize for the CC organization at every given opportunity. One lecturer will stop overweight women in department stores and urge them to join CC. Another calls every member of her class once during the weekend to check that none is cheating. When one lecturer sees any of her members gorging herself at a restaurant, she will send a note to the offender which says, "The CC fairy is watching you." Needless to say, the sinning CC member usually leaves the restaurant swiftly in blushing confusion.

CC knows that this type of behavior is regarded by members as caring and deep interest, albeit non CC'ers might feel such behavior is quite unnecessary interference in a person's private life. CC members are usually lonely and depressed people who are reaching out for companionship and authoritarian instruction. CC has a "hot-line" with a recorded message so that members who are tempted to falter and cheat may call the hot-line and hear a two-minute admonition on not cheating combined with promises as to what rewards await the CC'er in her new body. CC members bring little gifts and mementoes to their lecturers. The lecturers attend their members' weddings, visit them in the hospital, and call their members on the telephone. One Carbohydrate Counter lecturer even went on vacation to Florida with three members of her class just to prove to these ladies that they could stay "on program" even while on vacation. She and her class members rented an apartment in Miami. The lecturer prepared meals using the blender, special CC cookbooks, extracts, and powdered milk she had lugged with her on the airplane. On arrival back in Chicago, the quartet went directly to their CC office and weighed in. Each one had lost six pounds during vacation.

Lecturers are paid a minimum lecture fee which varies from region to region, but their real payoff comes from the doglike devotion of each member. Lecturers spend hours preparing the lectures, looking for visual aids, poring over their handbook, and attending lecturer workshops.

Lecturers become "stars" and they perform three, four, and five times a week. Their hours of work pay dividends in ego boosts. Loud laughter, giggles, and a continual buzzing undertone fill the room. When a nerve ending is struck, members react with laughter, although they are close to tears. When a lecturer is particularly funny, some members laugh so hard they begin to cry or

cannot stop laughing and have to leave the room. Borderline hysteria greeted this one lecturer's performance.

I like to take different roles and playact for my members. One evening after everyone had been weighed, I
changed my clothes and dressed up as a little girl. I had
ribbons in my hair, had a Raggedy Ann doll hanging
from my hand, and sucked on a big lollipop.

I walked up the aisle and people just gasped to see me.
I talked with a liddle girl lithp. I said that Momma used
to be so unhappy when she was taking those funny
green pills, but she was thin. Finally Daddy told her to
throw away the bottle or he would leave us and she
then got fat. Momma and I went to the movies one day
and she got stuck in the theater seat and then hit the
man with her purse who tried to pull her out. Momma
cried one day when her zipper got stuck on a new dress
when we were going to a weddin' and then Daddy told
her that she was too damned *fat*.

The performance continued with a recitation of Momma's problems which were obviously all the same difficulties of the audience, for the lecturer's drama was accompanied by hoots, snorts, and chuckles. The lecturer, Zelda,
received prolonged applause at the end of her Monday
performance and her fame spread. Telephones began ringing amongst CC members. For the Tuesday and Wednesday
shows, class size swelled. Class members from Monday
came Tuesday *and* Wednesday. Tuesday club members

caught the Wednesday performance. Other lecturers came to see if they could copy Zelda's role. The area manager invited Zelda to repeat her star performance for other area lecturers at a large workshop. (CC can be an amateur variety night more than a diet club.)

After they have been softened up by jokes, funny stories, barbed witticisms, and assorted visual aids, CC members hear their lecturer's fat story. CC members listen as their thin (formerly fat) lecturer recounts her sins.

> Peanut butter is my downfall. I love peanut butter with a passion. I can't stand to have it around the house. My kids are thin and they want to have peanut butter sandwiches. So I keep the peanut butter on a shelf in the garage in a box. Sometimes I get half crazy for peanut butter so I go out to the garage, climb up on a ladder, open the box, and unscrew the lid of the peanut butter. There I am in the garage smelling the peanut butter. I'm good. Don't get me wrong. Since I joined CC I haven't had a bite of peanut butter. But, oh God, I love to at least smell it.
>
> (twenty-nine-year-old female lecturer)

However, for CC lectures one subject is taboo—sex. Lecturers are warned that they are not to "talk dirty"; therefore, sex is a forbidden topic. CC recognizes that sex problems are often the basis for overweight. Some women eat because they dislike sex. Others overeat because they are married to impotent or uninterested husbands. Even though the husbands may be uninterested in sex because they are in bed beside an unappetizing lump of flesh, that is immaterial. Rather than completely uncork all the hidden psychoses of their members, Carbohydrate Counters wants only to treat symptoms lightly. A symptom may be that the woman is "mad" at her husband; but when the discussion gets too intimate, it is immediately cut off. However, members are anxious to talk about their sex lives, particularly at the weighing-in ceremony. They whisper to the clerk questions about whether or not fish is an aphrodisiac. They tell the lecturer in confidence that their sex lives have improved dramatically and that it must be due to the green vegetables they are eating. The lecturer nods her head in agreement and forgoes the temptation to tell members that they are probably more sexy because they are thinner.

Mutual confession and trading secrets help cement lecturer and member together in the bonds of CC.

When a member has reached her goal weight she is rewarded with a tiny pin and is expected to say a few words upon her "graduation." Invariably, the CC'er will give a little speech in which she bursts into tears and profusely, hiccupingly thanks her dear lecturer for all "her help and encouragement."

At times this "help and encouragement" take some rather strange forms. Lecturers will swear, yell, scream, and unmercifully berate a member who has gained. When a whole class has gained and not lost, I have seen lecturers pound the table and burst into tears, seemingly taking this weight gain as a personal insult.

These antics seem to work. CC members love their lecturers. CC members have found a haven for loneliness.

Even if the lecturer rages and raves, at least *someone* cares. Woe upon any substitute lecturer. Class-lecturer attachment can prove to be nearly pathological, as one area supervisor reports.

> We know we're in big trouble when we have to move a lecturer or when the lecturer regains her weight and we have to pull her out of her classes. We get hate mail, crank telephone calls, and threats from the classes. The classes think that their lecturer is the Virgin Mary and walks on water. One time we even got stink bombs set off in front of the office and received calls threatening our lives. The best ones are the members who have lost weight and they call up threatening to put back all the weight and make CC look ridiculous. The question really is who is ridiculous and who is crazy.
>
> (forty-three-year-old area supervisor, female)

Sometimes when area managers move a lecturer from one class to another or prohibit an overweight lecturer from giving classes until she loses weight, the lecturer will resign in a huff. Scab organizations have sprung up throughout the country formed by disaffected CC lecturers. CC makes its lecturers sign a sworn statement that they will not work for any other diet club for at least one year after leaving CC's employ. However, most of these scab groups are held in the former CC lecturer's home and members are sworn to secrecy. I visited one of these groups and the former CC lecturer told me how she had lost her weight through CC, had become a wildly popular lecturer, regained ten of her thirty-five pounds, and was removed from class until she lost weight. Unable to face her classes for shame and also unable to lose ten pounds, she telephoned some former class members and invited them to join her in a nonofficial CC class in her home.

> CC was my whole life. I lectured four times a week and all my friends were CC'ers. People used to stop me in the grocery store or on the street and talk to me about CC. I decided that I was making a lot of money for CC and that I could do just as well for people in my own home. Besides, I was tired of having to endure all their silly rules and all the petty fighting.

Numerous rules and much backstabbing are everyday occurrences in CC organization. Clerks, weigh-in clerks, lecturers, area managers, and regional supervisors all quarrel and fight with each other constantly. There are several reasons why CC staff squabble. The majority of employees are females who worked full-time only for a few years before marriage—often fifteen or so years prior to employment with CC. Thus, they have not learned proper office deportment, responsibility, compromise, or respect for a hierarchical chain of command. Queen of the kitchen, autocrat of the car pool, four-times-a-week star of the CC follies, CC lecturers brook no criticism. CC employees who are former housewives react violently and indeed hysterically to any suggestions for improvement.

Also, CC rules are regulations that encourage spying and tattletelling. CC handbooks for clerks, scale assistants, and lecturers advise that any breach of CC rules is to be reported to the office immediately. CC knows that it is dealing with sometimes foolish and often overemotional women who may or may not turn up for class and who may or may not behave appropriately. In order to maintain any semblance of order, the office staff stands ready to fill in for absent clerks or lecturers. Sometimes lecturers or clerks have violent quarrels in front of their classes and class members report these incidents to the home office. Some lecturers are highly unstable. Some have been known to preach hellfire and brimstone sermons of retribution, telling class members, "God will strike you dead if you don't follow program." Obviously in cases such as these, the main office ought to be called.

But CC employees seem to take a perverse delight in reporting each other to the office. These women enjoy cutting each other to pieces. It seems that the higher the education, the higher the husband's status, the better groomed the employee, or the more popular the lecturer, the more clerks and assistants complain. One lecturer finally gave up in disgust and left CC.

I couldn't take the way that I was treated. I worked for CC really as a hobby. It was fun and I enjoyed it. Then there were all these strange complaints from my clerks and assistants. My clothes were wrong; I had been seen wearing blue jeans; my tallies were incorrect; and God only knows what all. Finally it all came out one day when one clerk looked at me and said, "You think you are so damned high and mighty just because your husband is a lawyer. We'll fix you. We'll run you out."

Sometimes lecturers find that the continual responsibility of being at a given place at a specific time every single week is simply too much. A housewife who has always had a reasonably flexible schedule—or a constantly interrupted and nonexistent schedule—is easily baffled by rigid timetables. How then can she stop being a CC lecturer and still maintain her ego? Obviously, she cannot admit that she is unable to assume responsibility, although that is the reason for her resignation. The female sick role is called into play. An assorted bag of female problems is unleashed as the excuse for not working. CC lecturers who want to stop working also fall prey to the malady of "nerves."

> Susie just couldn't keep up with her classes. Her nerves bothered her a great deal. She was a wonderful lecturer and everyone adored her. She began to fall down on the job but it wasn't her fault—it was her "nerves."
>
> (thirty-year-old lecturer supervisor)

However, the frequency with which CC'ers erupt into tears and even hysteria cannot be attributed only to "nerves." Every CC lecture meeting that I attended ended up with at least two members of the group weeping. Perhaps years and years of diet pills have taken their toll in emotional stability. Perhaps women who have taken amphetamines for years are unable to withstand normal stresses and strains. Also, CC'ers are constant dieters. Often CC lecturers do not take their own advice about dieting. Several admitted to me that they had put on weight during a vacation and were starving for several days in order to peel the weight off and not be removed from classes for overweight. Starvation equals short tempers. In addition, CC lecturers often return to their diet pills to lose weight, even though diet pills are strictly forbidden on CC program. Strung out on pills, these CC employees magnify insignificant incidents into gigantic traumas—and then quit in anger.

Staff turnover varies from region to region, but all over the country outbursts and recriminations seem to be the rule and not the exception. CC has a rule that only CC members can be hired. Therefore, secretaries, file clerks, and switchboard operators in the main office are also fighting the battle of the bulge with its concomitant tantrums.

It is unfair to report only on highly neurotic and disturbed CC employees, for even though tempers flare and tears flow, CC lecturers are able to lead many members to the nirvana of thinness. One area manager recalled how she devoted more time to her CC classes than to her own family.

> If you only knew what I put my family through when I first started being a CC lecturer. I thought that I could save the whole world personally. I gave my telephone number out and told my classes to call me any time of the day or night. And brother, they sure did. I used to yell at my kids unmercifully to make them shut up when a CC'er called. My oldest son has a pronounced

stutter and the doctor says it's because I was so mean to him when I started working for CC.

(forty-four-year-old lecturer)

There are no adequate data concerning the success rate of diet clubs in general or CC in particular. Dieters are fickle, as Mead Johnson of Metrecal fame found out to their million-dollar sorrow. It may be that the diet-club fad has run its course. Dieters have gone from gizmos with flashing lights to weight belts to caramel candy to methylcellulose to cyclamate to saccharin and back again. The weight-control business is a good money-making, profit-garnering business because dieters are capricious. From an evangelical point of view, CC wants thin people. From the standpoint of profits, the yo-yo syndrome of the professional dieter is a big dollar sign in the eyeballs of CC executives.

CC does retrain many people into regimented, well-balanced eating, although they don't understand nutrition. The CC organization has a better rate of success than the average doctor's 2 percent rate. Yet no adequate data exist telling us what the dropout rate is among CC dieters. As a general rule of thumb, area supervisors estimate that 30 percent of dieters drop out of CC meetings after two sessions. Of the remaining 70 percent, nearly all lose some weight (that is, two pounds or more), while maybe 30 percent reach their goal. Of that 30 percent, we don't know how many had only ten pounds to lose and how many over a hundred. Nevertheless, CC clubs are phenomenally profitable. They do not sell a profit, they merchandise dreams.

Everyone achieves some kind of satisfaction from the

association with Carbohydrate Counters. Fat members have an evening out and free entertainment. Members who lose weight reach goal and maybe even become lecturers. Lecturers become vaudeville stars and are idolized by their fans. Clerks and assistants earn a few dollars and spy on lecturers. Above all, CC makes a profit. Three dollars here. Five dollars there. CC rings up the cash registers unceasingly, week after month after year.

Carbohydrate Counters or any diet club will always be a success. While diet clubs advertise their wares, the "thin" message is everywhere. Ladies' magazines offer a new magic diet. Paris invents a new slim silhouette. Thin is in. Fat is out. Ten pounds overweight is bad. Twenty pounds is wicked. Fifty or more pounds is positively evil. Think of the agony that the thin society produces for nearly everyone. She who has broad hips is forever cursed. She who has a pudgy chin is worthless. She who can't fit into a size 7 dress is not socially acceptable. These motifs bombard women (and men too) whenever they read a popular magazine or watch commercial TV. Heroines are never fat!

So in combination with a diet club—or as antidote to—or as adjunct to a sedentary office job—the next step is the health club.

3 The Body Shop

Diet club, pills, or quack doctors to no avail, Ms. Fat
America has one other avenue to lose weight effortlessly
and quickly—the reducing salon. Newspaper advertising
and magazines portray lithe young ladies in black leotards
under banners stating:

YOU CAN BE BEAUTIFUL AND SHAPELY IN JUST TEN DAYS!

or

IF YOU ARE A SIZE 14 *NOW*—YOU CAN BE A SIZE 10

IN JUST 31 DAYS!!!

or

OUR MACHINES DO THE WORK FOR YOU

ALL YOU DO IS LOSE INCHES!

Tempted by the promise of a "lovelier you" and a more shapely body in just a few days, the gullible customer-to-be calls the salon for her "free" or "reduced price" appointment.

Let us take a look at the reducing salon and the methods by which a customer is enticed to sign a contract. Keep in mind, however, that we are speaking in broad generalities about practices found in an estimated 1,500 reducing salons, health spas, health studios, and exercise salons in the United States which earn approximately $350 million per year. There are many reputable clubs, organizations, recreation centers, YMCA's and YWCA's that cater to Mr. and Mrs. Average who seek to keep physically fit. Given publicity over heart attacks, high blood pressure, and the evils of the sedentary overweight life which mean in essence a shortened life span, more and more Americans are jogging, swimming, and exercising to keep off flab and get the cardiovascular system back in shape. That's good. That's healthy and sensible. As a matter of fact, there is something good and sensible and healthy about wanting to get rid of bulges and ripples of fat. Aesthetically minded people can be healthy people too. What we refer to in this chapter is the undercurrent of fad, fraud, deception, and deliberate misinformation presented to a too-gullible public.

For those who want an easy rule of thumb, here's one to begin with. The more Spartan the decor, the less likely it is that the owners/managers will rip you off. Decor varies according to whether the organization advertises itself as a health studio, health spa, or reducing salon. Health studios are no-nonsense institutions run by devotees in the Bernarr Macfadden health-food tradition. The body fit is more important than the body beautiful, although fitness and beauty are generally equated. Health-studio customers and owners compare serious notes on vitamins, health foods, wheat germ, blackstrap molasses, and organic foods. Most of these products are also for sale in the reception room of the health studio—at outrageous prices. Located downtown in deteriorating sections of the city, presided over by burly Scandinavian Amazons, the health studios reek of liniment and foot powder. However, with the advent of fast-buck reducing salons in the suburbs, health studios are slowly disappearing from the scene.

Health spas are much more flamboyant than reducing salons. For example, one health spa flanks its huge ten-foot-wide double door entranceway with seven-foot male and female figures holding enormous flaming torches, while a syndicated reducing salon covers its windows with looped, lush, swagged Austrian valances and only a discreet brass nameplate informs the public what goes on inside. On entering, the visitor is immediately struck by the basic requirement of all salons—a chandelier. In over thirty visits to as many salons and health spas in five cities, I found not one without a crystal chandelier in the reception area. Actually, the price of treatments is directly related to the number of crystal chandeliers found in the salon.

Chandeliers aside, most salons are decorated in a crazy mixture of early Sear's kitsch, neo-bordello, early Holiday Inn, and Texas saloon revival. Walls are decorated with fuzzy art-nouveau wallpaper and adorned with gilt-edged and cupid-bedecked mirrors. Mirrors are everywhere: large mirrors, small mirrors, framed mirrors, and worst of all, in the exercise room, mirrors that completely cover walls from floor to ceiling.

Peeking at her reflection in these many mirrors, the visitor glumly realizes that she is a walking testimonial for the ''before'' pictures in newspaper ads, while the nubile, shiny-haired instructor in her black leotard is living, vibrant proof of a beautiful ''after.'' This creature of loveliness hangs up the customer's coat, asks her to change into leotards and then come to the exercise room. Now the shell game begins.

Under glaring, harsh fluorescent lights in a dazzling mirrored hall, the unsuspecting customer is calmly measured by her instructor-guide. Nervously she awaits the verdict about thigh, calf, hip, and waist measurements. She already knows that her bustline is far too small. All American women know that their bustlines are too tiny. The instructor tells the customer to stand up straight and not bend down to look at the tape. There is very good reason for this admonishment because on the first visit to any salon, measurements are taken with an exceedingly loose tape. Thus within a week or ten days, on being remeasured with tautly held tape, the customer finds to her delight that she has lost an inch here, a half-inch there, and a quarter of an inch someplace else. To test this fraud, one day in Chicago I went to five different salons, and found my waist and hip measurements varied by two inches—plus or minus. Hopefully I was not gaining or losing inches as I went up and down the Loop and Michigan Avenue, but apparently something was happening.

After recording the potential client's measurements with only an occasionally raised eyebrow or pursed lips, the instructor pauses a moment, makes a few swift calculations on the card, and then shows the customer the card once more. Voilà! Hocus pocus!! There written in indelible ball-point ink for all the world to see are two columns: one with today's date shows the customer's measurements, and the other, labeled six weeks away, shows what she *will* measure. Thus forty-inch hips will shrink to a teeny thirty-six inches, and a tubby thirty-inch waist will whittle down to a tiny twenty-four inches. How will this be done? With these marvelous machines, of course. Bedazzled by thoughts of a new svelte self, the customer begins her Alice-in-Wonderland free trip through the land of magic machines.

Leading the customer through the salon, the instructor spends more time demonstrating the passive exercisers. The idea here, of course, is to entice the prospect by emphasizing no-fuss, no-effort exercising. Even though salons vary according to whether or not they include extra-special services such as saunas, swimming pools, massage tables, facial and pedicure experts, beauty parlors, and whirlpool therapy, most chain or local exercise or health studios have the usual standard assortment of exercise machines and their customer pitch is remarkably similar. While instructors introduce their would-be clients to lo-rollers, hi-rollers, belt-hip massagers, and stationary bicycles, they explain that these machines "break down fat by stimulating blood circulation." Some machines are touted as "burning up the calories released by vibrating machines." The athletic and bosomy instructor spends very little time illustrating the ballet bar or pull-down machines which require more effort and concentration. As a matter of fact, she only casually mentions the exercise class which takes place every hour and half-hour.

So after the swift and nontiring tour, the visitor is ushered into the office of the owner/manager, who begins his supersales pitch. Owner/managers are usually greasy, sleazy, oily, lecherous men who constantly lick their lips and look with lust upon their female clients. Rather than being embarrassed by such unctuous attention, the client is rather titillated. Squirming in her too-tight clothes, conscious of her bulges and lumps, she is pathetically grateful for his oozing attention and more than eager to sign on the dotted line. What does she sign?

She often signs a long-term contract with tiny print stating that the owner can sue her or garnishee 22 percent of her wages should she not continue with the program. That is, if the customer moves, becomes ill, or, as usually happens, just simply loses interest or becomes bored, she is still iron-clad-bound to her contract. Even if she is shrewd enough to insist on the advertised "special rate," at the end of the specified period of visits the owner/managers often pull the old bait-and-switch trick on her. At the end of the ten advertised special-rate sessions, when the customer concludes that she is not as gorgeous as she wants to be or was promised to be by the misleading advertising, she is told that ten sessions are simply not enough for "her problem."

Bedazzled by the thought of having a "personalized exercise program all her very own," she is easily persuaded to sign up for ten more sessions. And ten more sessions. And more and more. Somehow *her* "after" never seems as wonderful as the newspaper advertisements. She rarely wises up to the fact that the "before" and "after" pictures are often faked with different lighting, different clothing, and sometimes even different people. Of course she will never look like the wonderful "after" picture, unless she has a whole studio of professional public relations experts doing a number for her. So customer after customer is bilked by false promises, false advertising, and shoddy business practices. The client is never told that she can be sued, harassed, and hounded for payment once she signs a contract. Gazing raptly at the shining chandeliers, thrilled by the male manager's attention, anxious to become beautiful in only six weeks, and overwhelmed by compliments, she signs on the dotted line above all that fine print. Such nice people couldn't be frauds.

The studio's apparent professionalism is another sham. Instructors are chosen because of their slender figures and not because of any professional training. The health clubs intimate that their instructors are only short of a graduate degree in physical education but the facts are usually contrary to this "impression." An ad that appeared in the *Washington Post* help-wanted section underscores the lack of training for figure salon instructors. Listed in the "sales" section of the classifieds, the ad proclaimed in part: "Our sales training program will teach you all you need to know to help yourself!" Under "Qualifications" were listed such things as owning a car, willingness to work nights and Saturdays, and having a good figure. No mention was made of a background in physical education or physiology.

Untrained instructors working on commission harangue their clients and sometimes lead them into dangerously strenuous sessions. One instructor whom I interviewed was very proud of her exercise "manual," which consisted of a loose-leaf notebook with exercises cut out of ladies' magazines pasted on the pages. Another admitted that her only training was taking an exercise class at the local Y, while yet another said her only training consisted of ballet lessons when she was five years old. Instructors generally are bored mannequins unable to get a job anywhere else who take this assignment in desperation. Often sneaking away to the ladies' washroom for a quick cigarette break, they spend more time talking to each other and gossiping on the telephone than with customers. Instructors can scarcely conceal their hatred of their clientele. In interviews, instructors sometimes referred to the customers as "pigs," "sweat-hogs," "cows," "elephants," and "dumb-dumbs." "Bitch" is such a common term it is nearly a form of endearment.

Instructors resent having to cater to the whims of bored, overweight, frustrated, and often nasty housewives. In many salons the warfare between instructors and clients breaks down into several categories: thin versus overweight, working versus nonworking women, young versus old, and beautiful versus ugly. All the secret fears of the overweight middle-aged housewife are unleashed by the presence of young, energetic, svelte, and cute instructors. But the instructors themselves can panic when they see their customers. They see their own future—three kids, thirty pounds, and fifteen years hence.

All is not woe. Some clients do lose weight and many lose inches. Their success and a word-of-mouth campaign are the best advertising a salon can have. Yet mixed up with the truth of lost inches is the myth of the salon.

TRUE: Regular exercise will tone and firm muscles.

FALSE: Exercise machines break down fatty tissue, stimulate blood circulation, and redistribute fatty deposits.

Nevertheless, satisfied customers chant about wonderful machines that redistribute fatty deposits or break down fat. Simply to admit to cutting down on calorie intake and increasing calorie expenditure would be admitting to previous sloth, so even newly thin customers must cloak their accomplishments in miraculous explanations. While diet is not emphasized, weekly weighing is. The client is expected to follow some reducing diet—supplied by the salon or by the customer. Many salons hand out "magic" diets consisting of high-protein, low-fat plans that once again are touted as mysterious calorie burners. In light of possible law suits, salons do not insist on dieting but only "suggest."

And so the ladies huff and puff, strain, bend, push, and jiggle their fat. A series of questionnaires administered to patrons of one salon, visits to thirty salons, interviews with twenty instructors from as many spas in five cities, have given me a perspective on exercise salons' patrons and practices.

One surprising result was that long-term members who had attended a salon for over a year had lost *less* weight and inches than those women who came to the salon for a brief period of time but who attended intensive sessions. That is, women who used the salon for the sole purpose of exercising and losing weight, lost weight faster and more efficiently than long-term members. It seems reasonable to conclude that women who use the salon as a kaffee-klatch gossip club are afraid to achieve success by losing inches because this will mean disengagement from their favorite spot.

This subconscious control over *not* losing weight was seen in the "Chubby Chart Incident" in one salon. Patrons were expected to fill out daily hour-by-hour reports on every morsel of food ingested and hand the charts to the instructor when returning to the salon. These Chubby Charts were to remind the chronic nibbler how much she was really eating and so act as effective curbs on those women who contended that they "don't eat a thing and still gain weight." Two instructors had asked their patrons to keep Chubby Charts which would be collected after Thanksgiving. *Every one* flatly refused to fill out her Chubby Chart. They were all quite straightforward in their explanations. All admitted that they were planning to overeat during Thanksgiving. One woman said, "I don't want anyone else to know how much I'm going to eat." Another said, "My God! My arm would fall off if I wrote down everything that I ate over Thanksgiving.'' These women are supposedly rational wives and mothers—women who pay good money to pound themselves at an exercise salon, women who are painfully aware of every calorie count for every bite of food: but still they coolly plan eating binges regardless of the consequences. At the same time, the interviews with patrons showed an incredible ambivalence. Most women said that they were adhering strictly to a diet but the *same* women admitted to snacking between meals; most said that they regularly ate candy; and half said that they served themselves large amounts of food and took second helpings. Yet it is logically contradictory to reconcile dieting with snacking, eating candy, and consuming bountiful helpings of rich foods.

While they admitted to overeating and overindulgence, many women were ingenious in explaining away any weight gain. Some blamed their overeating on other people: ''My neighbor brought over a pie and I just had to taste it''; or, ''It's all my husband's fault, he makes me eat.'' Others recognized that they were too weak to resist external cues: ''I wish they would quit showing those commercials with all that good food''; or, ''That ice-cream parlor speaks to me every time I go by the door.'' Some of the excuses were bizarre to say the least: ''The weather always makes me retain water''; ''I had sex last night with my husband and it always makes me gain weight.''

In spite of candidly confessing to planning overeating binges, most patrons are unable to face the fact that they overeat and underexercise. While they lie about themselves and their own lack of self-control, they are ever eager to criticize other patrons. As each woman bounces and pedals furiously on one machine or another, she keeps an eagle eye trained on friends and acquaintances twisting and pounding to her left and right.

Trading gossip and choosing every opportunity to insult, deride, tease, and otherwise degrade their neighbor bouncing and jiggling on the next machine, patrons harpoon each other. Each woman spies on the others, hoping to see increases in girth rather than decreases. Instead of concentrating on their own rippling fat, they delight in discovering the sins of other patrons. Of course, the confessional approach elicits admissions of sin on the neighbor's part. When one woman publicly announces that she fell off the wagon, her neighbors to her left and right recount their sins of backsliding as well. One woman will start off a train of disclosures with a simple statement like, "Oh dear! I'm really ashamed of myself because I really had too many drinky-poohs over the weekend." A chorus answers, "Yes, yes, me too." "How terrible." "I know I gained ten pounds from my sister-in-law's cooking." Like a line of benign elephants they croon and sympathize with each other. Evil days will befall the woman who coolly announces that she stuck to her diet, has lost weight, feels wonderful, and bounces from machine to machine like a lithe teen-ager. Success is not tolerated easily amongst the salon crowd.

A favorite pastime is to tear the instructor to shreds. While ideally the instructor should be an inspirational example of successful dieting and healthful exercise, she is a constant thorn in the clients' chubby sides. Thus one way

patrons relieve their guilt over not dieting and not exercising is to gossip unmercifully about their instructors. Of
course, the instructors' hostility toward their clientele
elicits some of this reaction, but it is a moot point as to who
hates whom more—instructor or client. Patrons are fixated
on the instructor's sex life, be she married or single. Obviously someone who looks as good as the leggy blond
instructor simply has to be immoral.

Clients hoarsely whisper *sotto voce* eager recitations
of their instructors' supposed sexual peccadilloes. Having
personally interviewed some instructors, I was amazed to
hear the scatalogical references that they suffered from their
clients. Vicious gossip is the order of the day at the reducing
salon. No wonder then that the instructor flees at the sight of
her enemies trudging glumly to the salon in black leotards
with even blacker lies to cast about.

But even more interesting to the salon devotees is the
instructor's appetite. In small cities, customers regale each
other with tales of how much they saw the instructor eating
at a local restaurant, how much food she was seen purchas-
ing at the grocery store, or how often she patronizes the
ice-cream-store-down-the-street. The instructor's gargan-
tuan appetite serves as *bona fide* evidence that she has
overactive glands and can consume mountains of food,
while her chunky customers have an overabundance of fat
cells, an underactive metabolism, and a lumpy body.

Patrons continually fabricate a pantheon of rationalizations to explain why they don't lose inches. But clear-
eyed observations of patrons in reducing salons reveal that
most customers exercise as little as possible and avoid it as

much as possible, even when paying money to have someone else force them to use machines and exercise! Their actions, in contrast to their excuses, uncover the truth. On the hour and half-hour, instructors gaily announced that the time had come for patrons to leave their machines and join in a fifteen-minute group-exercise session. Moaning, groaning, mumbling curses, and vocalizing porcine squeals, patrons would slowly space themselves around the room. Some women would pretend to join in but actually would hide themselves behind a large piece of equipment to conceal themselves from the instructor. Others would faint-heartedly bend and stretch to avoid any outright criticism from the instructor but also so feebly as to insure that no benefit would take place. Still others would sit cross-legged on the floor and belligerently refuse to take part in the class because they were soooo exhausted from the passive exercise machines. That would leave only a few valiant souls doggedly following the instructor's commands. Actually in some classes only the instructor seemed to be straining herself and really exercising, while the rest of the class goofed off or went on strike. It was too reminiscent of those painful physical education classes that I struggled through in high school.

But just like high school, every salon or studio exercise class has its own clown—a woman who makes cutting remarks about the instructor, or who pretends to die a miserably gasping death from exhaustion. One woman I observed tried to do some exercises and then collapsed in a size 16 heap on the floor, moaning out loud that her back was broken, her lungs had collapsed, all her muscles had snapped. The rest of the class giggled excitedly at her display of temperament and independence. Since the instructor was a young girl of eighteen or twenty, she found it awkward to reprimand a woman some twenty years older than herself who was acting like a two-year-old. Caught between the demands of maintaining order and overstepping the bounds of age-defined decorum, the instructor attempted to jolly the recalcitrant sinner into place. "Now, now, Mrs. Adams, it just can't be that bad," she cajoled. Mrs. Adams screamed that it was indeed *VERY, VERY* bad. And the banter continued. Usually the tubby customer wins her battle: The instructor retires from the fray with a grimace of disgust, the class has a few moments of rest during their supposedly strenuous exercise break, and everyone is satisfied. After flopping on the floor like beached whales, customers then headed toward their favorite machines—the passive exercisers. One woman proclaimed loudly, "This thing really turns me on," while others agreed in chorus that the vibrator belt gave them some sort of thrill. The vibrator seems to do little more than provide a masturbationlike sensation.

Actually, it would take fifteen minutes on the vibrator belt every day for a year for a person to lose just one pound of fat, and there is no indication that fat is shifted from one place to another by the vibrating machines. But information like this is not widely known. Salon ladies are convinced that the machines will perform magic tricks. Machines will bounce away the fat. Vibrators will do the trick. If not vibrators, then magic packs and quickie wraps.

Some pseudo-spas capitalize on the idea of losing

weight with *absolutely no effort whatsoever.* Throughout the United States, salons have been touting the wrapping technique, by which the customer is tightly bound and wrapped in a series of gauze bandages until she resembles a pudgy mummy. Tottering and weaving she is led to a tub where she and her gauze mummy bandages are soaked in a magic-secret-not-to-be-divulged formula and then popped into a plastic suit. She lies in her plastic suit, sometimes under heat lamps, for a few hours and then is unzipped, unwrapped, and remeasured. Voilà! Once again the impossible has happened! For an exorbitant fee she has lost a few inches. Of course, the customer does not lose these inches permanently but has to return again and again for more treatments. The Better Business Bureau and the American Medical Association warn repeatedly that these treatments are dangerous to the health of women with varicose veins, phlebitis, cardiac condition, or high blood pressure.

Still quacks persist. Still women seek beauty through sorcery. Unable to accept the fact that a balanced diet and regular exercise will slowly accomplish what they want so much—curves and no lumps—they flock to salon, spa, and studio hearkening to the siren call of false advertising. Cash registers clank. Bank accounts increase. Fat is big business.

Some women thought that nirvana had arrived with the discovery of the electric muscle stimulator. Women attached pads to fatty parts of their bodies, attached wires to the pads, and then turned a switch activating the wires. Electrical impulses were then sent to the muscles and the muscles jumped like crazy. Relaxicizor led the muscle stimulator business for nearly twenty-one years, sold instruments ranging from $100 to $400, and grossed nearly $40 million. After years of threats, years of Relaxicizor's supposed compliance, years of fudging and years of pussyfooting, the FDA finally went to court in 1966. After four years of delays and a half million dollars in time and effort, the decree was handed down. The judge ruled that Relaxicizor was not only worthless but actually a menace. He declared that the machine was capable of inducing heart failure and had the power to add to "gastrointestinal, orthopedic, muscular, neurological, kidney, gynecological and pelvic disorders." Moreover, he said it very possibly aggravated "epilepsy, hernia, multiple sclerosis, spinal fusion, tubo-ovarian abscess, ulcers and varicose veins." It was really not the judge's decision that scared away the Relaxicizor customers but just the fact that the judge was mean enough to forbid the sale of any more Relaxicizors. So rushing to fill the gap left by Relaxicizor came Sauna Jeans, Sauna Belts, and Trim Jeans.

An energetic Californian, Jack Feather, claims to be the father of the inflatable belt, or inflatable Sauna Jeans craze. It seems that Jack Feather used to wrap the lady exercisers who patronized his chain of health studios in Ace bandages. Lo and behold, wrapped lady exercisers lost inches more quickly than unwrapped lady exercisers. Jack Feather added a rubber cover, then a plastic cover, and the Sauna Belt came into being. Post office investigators moved in to charge Jack Feather with fraud but were unable to prove their case. But, on the other hand, the post office did win its case against Sauna Shorts. There seems to be no rhyme nor reason for these conflicting decisions except that perhaps the case against Sauna Shorts was prepared more carefully after the Sauna Belt case had just been lost. The post office built its case on a comparative study of thirty prison inmates who all followed the same exercise program, but half of whom wore Sauna Shorts and half did not. There was no difference recorded in girth and no spot reduction noted between the group who had worn Sauna Shorts and those who had not.

No matter what the FDA or post office or AMA or Better Business Bureau or learned judges decide, women still fall for every kind of gimmickry, quackery, and tomfoolery around. But the relation between the con artist and victim is terrifyingly intimate. The victim is willing accomplice to the con artist. Why not? She is bombarded on every side by newspaper, magazine, and television advertising—all telling her repeatedly that she has to be thin, must be thin, is most assuredly a social failure if she is fat, and offering a magic way to become thin. Whether slickies like *Cosmopolitan* and *Vogue* or pulps like *True Confessions* and *Real Romances,* the message is hot. Buy my product and become thin.

Just casually glancing through the pages of women's magazines, any average Martian would come to the immediate conclusion that American women are weight and breast obsessed. Here are but a few samples of screaming headline advertising banners:

"I actually ate 6 full meals a day and lost 69 pounds of ugly fat in only 30 days."

"I lost 61 pounds of excess fat by just relaxing in my bathtub."

———————

"Amazing Slimo for $6.95."

———————

"Trim your waistline in 3 days for $3.98."

———————

"Body-wrap for $19.95."

———————

"Insta-slim girdle for men and women $6.99."

———————

"Melt Your Bulging Tummy Away for $9.95."

———————

"Do You Suffer from the Globbies?"

———————

"Skinny Suit $12.95."

———————

For five dollars here, two dollars there, or twenty dollars someplace else, health, fame, beauty, and success can be the reader's. Nowhere else in one fell swoop can you find the perverted American dream in all its tarnished glory except on the pages of women's magazines. While we indict American advertising for its utter irresponsibility, we must also excoriate American women for their gullibility. These women accept the stereotype of the beautiful dumb broad. To be successful and happy a woman has to be beautiful. Being beautiful in America means being blond, thin-hipped, flat-tummied, and big-boobed.

I made an analysis of advertising in ten women's magazines. I found that although nearly 60 percent of the ads were concerned with beauty, 6 percent of the advertisements had something to do with bust improvement. Indeed the sheer *number* of ads for bust improvement is overwhelming.

It's fascinating to note that even the sexy slickies like *Cosmopolitan* feature a bosomy model in a low-cut gown on the front cover. What this implies I'm not too sure, but at least we find that big-chested women are admired by *Cosmo*'s staff. Perhaps the model bought a bust-improver product like Mark Eden's, the leader in the bust-improvement field. One typical quote from its ads reads:

> "I never dreamed that after four children I would ever regain my bustline, but after just six weeks, I have gone from a 32A to a 36C."
>
> Mrs. D. T., Texas

In the past few years, Beauti-Brest has been creeping up on Mark Eden. Beauti-Brest is an ingenious device that hooks up to the water faucet and to an electric whoogie. By turning the water on full blast and also plugging in the little electric stimulator, the contour cup "stimulates breast tissue." You bet it does. While Beauti-Brest reports gains of up to six inches in one treatment, you can accomplish much the same result by hitting yourself on the breast with a board. Any tissue that endures stress or trauma will become engorged. So much for Beauti-Brest.

Ms. America remains convinced that by spending a few dollars for a magic pill or an inflatable plastic body suit, she will get rid of her extra flab and become happy. If Ms.

Average only had a few thousand dollars she could fulfill her secret dream.

Ms. Average America has a recurring fantasy—to spend a week or two at a luxury spa. Elizabeth Arden's Main Chance and Golden Door and others of the ever proliferating luxury spa business located in Mexico, Switzerland, Bermuda, and Yugoslavia cater to jet-setters, movie stars, and ultra-chic *doyennes.* Ms. Average moons over the pages of *Vogue, Women's Wear Daily,* and *Harper's Bazaar* which breathlessly tout the infinite pleasures of every spa. Drooling over every paragraph, Ms. Suburbia finds sisterhood in the thought that the beautiful people pay up to and above a thousand dollars per week for the same dream of instant beauty.

Dressed in pink terry-cloth exercise suits, women (and some men) submit to hours of bumping, straining, pounding, and low-calorie meals. Looking like pink pudgy teddy bears, the not-so-beautiful but oh-so-rich bend and strain, soak and sweat under the gimlet eyes of their wardens. A luxury spa is a luxury prison. Inmates are under twenty-four-hour surveillance lest they cheat and break training with a martini or a chocolate mousse. Client-inmates are wakened early for a constant round of exercise classes, massages, swimming pool exercises, saunas, and gourmet but calorieless meals. It is comforting to know that even though beautiful people pay enormous amounts to rid themselves of minuscule lumps of fat, they too have weak spirits. Many are the tales told of clients who smuggle in food and liquor in an effort to offset the Spartan regime.

(Many too are the tales told of such luxury spas as being more drying-out spots for lushes than reducing spas.)

One friend of mine has a tale that I consider hysterically funny—but she doesn't. Evelyn's dream of spending a sybaritic week at Elizabeth Arden's was always curtailed by her limited bank account. Overweight and somewhat overwrought, she finally saw her dream come true in an ad for a salon that was ridiculously cheap and yet promised both miracles and fun. She called the toll-free number and asked if there were recreational facilities such as tennis and swimming. She was told that indeed there were and they expected her to come and partake of their luxury atmosphere. Delighted, she made reservations and drove up to the appointed spot. Alas, the building was rather Charles Addamsish, complete with a ghoulish mad doctor with a thick Austrian accent, who Evelyn contends was an ex-Nazi guard.

When she arrived, the management told her that swimming was in the outdoor community pool in a town some ten miles away; tennis likewise was in the far-off town. But the best was yet to come. The mad doctor from Buchenwald asked Evelyn if she had ever fasted for long. "Fasted!" Evelyn gasped. "Where are the gourmet diet recipes and lovely little lunches that you advertise?" She was then informed that there really were no little gourmet lunches or little gourmet anything, or any food for that matter. Strict fasting was the order of the day, and pounds would immediately melt away. That explained why the cost was so low as well.

Evelyn's pounds did melt away but some of her sanity did too for a while. Her sister recounts that Evelyn would call at midnight or three o'clock in the morning, hallucinating and crying and screaming about terrible people and torture. The sister thought the whole thing a marvelous joke and kept encouraging poor starving, hallucinating Evelyn to stay at the spa. Evelyn admits to losing some thirty pounds and her memories of starvation fade as she recounts how she entered an upper New York State torture camp and survived.

Evelyn is no different from most of us who will continuously search for Beauty with a capital *B*. And beauty attained effortlessly and instantly. But no matter. The ultimate is the pseudo-scientific pseudo-medical spa with weird and wonderful concoctions, injections, pills, draughts, and potions. Wild and outlandish mixtures promise Ponce de León's dream. Doses are made from chicken embryos, unborn lambs, sea kelp, and God only knows what else. Why, it is even rumored that the Pope himself patronizes one such spa!

However, such pleasures are beyond the budget of Ms. Average Housewife, although she may pause and daydream about the faint possibility of entering these hallowed halls of beauty. She has to be content with her neighborhood or suburban spa—not one in Bermuda. Rather than surrendering her body to a daily massage with her own personal masseuse, she has to be content to lose inches with a vibrator belt, then plastic inflatable pantaloons, if not bloomers, then weight belts and maybe that wrapping salon over the freeway, or maybe that box of methylcellulose wafers or maybe . . .

Or maybe she'll just get her hair done. Getting your hair done is an American institution and the best way of feeling better quickly.

4 Beastly Beautician

From birth to death, hairdressing is an integral feature of most women's lives. Often a woman remembers her first visit to a salon at age two, when her mother plunked her down on top of several telephone books and an unwilling stylist cut baby's hair. From then on, many women are caught in a never ending round of visits to the beauty salon. Milestone events ranging from first communion to proms to wedding day all depend on beauty-parlor appointments and an appropriate hairdo for each occasion. Women sometimes even fight labor pains to get their hair properly styled before checking in at the hospital. Passing years are noted by tints to cover the gray, cuts to appear more youthful, and blue rinses to lighten white hair. Some women state in their wills which hairdresser they want to perform the last magic rites.

With such faithful clientele, no wonder that hairdressing is a multibillion-dollar business. Beauty shop receipts reached $4.7 billion in 1975 and may reach $7.3 billion in 1980. Two out of three American women own at least one wig; more than $1 billion was spent on wigs in 1970, and nearly a quarter of a million dollars on styling and cleaning wigs. In addition, nearly one-third of all American women tint or bleach their hair. Over a third of all American women patronize a beauty shop every week.

Hairdressing is a lucrative "profession" for a high-school dropout or college graduate. With hard work and good management a shop owner can make $35,000 per year. A married woman with children can work part-time and on weekends for extra money. A politically savvy male beautician can attain prominence via competitions, become a judge, open a school, and rake in close to $100,000 per year. But most hairdressers don't look that far ahead; they just need to learn a trade.

The type of beauty school chosen by the prospective beautician forever stamps and molds his or her career. There are Ivy League swish professional hair-styling schools and shoddy fly-by-night swindlers that prey on unsuspecting young people. Even though some states claim to monitor beauty schools, all too often these schools are shabby con jobs. I have visited many kinds and types of schools and the (unfortunately) typical school is a hole-in-the-wall organization with comings and goings of customer and student. The interesting thing is the manner in which the owner can make money.

School owners receive student fees, yet students sign a contract which often states that even if the student doesn't complete the course—for whatever reason: illness or boredom or lack of interest—the student or parent cosigner still has to pay the school owner full tuition. In addition, the school owner makes money from the customers who flock to the schools hoping to obtain an inexpensive hairdo or permanent. Also the school owner buys supplies at massive discounts and then sells the supplies to the students at a markup. Not bad all the way round. Usually beauty schools are located in low-rent areas, and, since there is no need for expensive beauty-shop decor, given the walk-in clientele, overhead costs are extremely low. But profits are high.

Customers certainly don't seem to mind the lack of amenities. Price wins out over comfort. There are usually large numbers of women of all ages, sizes, and even economic strata waiting to have their hair done for one or two dollars. Price wins out over worries that the cut will be ragged or the permanent frizzy. The young student and the old lady pensioner, the harried mother on a budget and the fellow beauty-school student are each willing to endure long waits and hit-or-miss service. Students themselves sometimes are leery of their customers, as one hairdresser remembered.

Migod! You can't imagine what those school customers were like. Some of them had lice and crud in their hair that made you want to throw up. Others were the grande dames who ordered you around like the school was Elizabeth Arden's or something. You learned to deal with the public all right because you learned to deal with the crummiest kind of public. I guess the ones that were the hardest to deal with were the house-wife types who desperately wanted to look nice for a party—and then when they didn't turn out gorgeous because an inexperienced kid had done her hair—then all hell broke loose.

Beauty school is a far cry from the discipline of high school and has more of a grade-school ambience. Inter-views with school owners show that discipline and theft are the two main problems in the school. Since the majority of girls (and the few boys) are high-school dropouts and have likely been truants, regular attendance is a painful problem. Since each state requires that a student attend beauty school for a specified number of hours (usually 1,500), strict attendance must be kept on each student. The students (and graduates) bitterly complain at being "docked" one hour for every portion of fifteen minutes late they arrive in the morning or come late from lunch. There is a dual purpose in this rigid punishment. First of all, the school owner quickly teaches students that tardiness will not be tolerated. And secondly, as a result of absences and tardiness, students remain in school for longer periods of time—like serfs or indentured servants. This misuse of power in order to have not-so-willing workers extends itself to the good student. In most states students are allowed to present themselves for hairdressing examinations at the discretion of the school director. That is, a student who has completed the required number of hours of classroom and practical instruction still needs permission of the school owner. Thus a competent student who has completed all the requirements and who has built up a reasonably steady clientele may not be allowed to go to the state exam for, say, six months. As the student increases her speed, she does more customers; as her work improves, she has more return customers; and all in all the school owner makes more money from tuition and customer fees.

Of course not all schools are rip-offs and not all school owners are unscrupulous, but complaints from working hairdressers were so constant, regardless of the section of the country I was interviewing in, that it does seem some more stringent regulations should be directed at these trade schools. For example, inspectors or state investigators should look into whether owner/student contracts are fraudulent, the treatment of students vis-à-vis attendance, the sanitary or unsanitary conditions of the shop, markup on beauty products, and teaching standards.

While most trade schools have some weak rules governing the competence of staff, beauty schools have little or none. Practicing beauticians have perpetuated the myth that beauty-school instructors are beauticians who could never make it in the hurly-burly beauty-shop world and so turned to teaching. Perhaps. As a matter of fact, the instructors didn't seem any more informed than their students. Most states require a minimal amount of knowledge of basic chemistry, some anatomy of face and head, and a slight knowledge of muscles and nerves for a facial and upper body massage. Students use antiquated textbooks and teachers engage in brief rote memorization of these sections. Since allergies, skin rashes, and serious burns may result from inadequate testing of bleaches, tints, or permanent wave solution, students should be given more up-to-date knowledge regarding dangers of beauty products. Even though serious charges may be leveled at cosmetic manufacturers, it is to the producers' credit that there are not more serious accidents every day in the beauty salons, especially since beauticians are so inadequately prepared.

Out-of-date textbooks teach pincurls and finger waving and ignore current modish methods of combing and styling. No wonder then that students complain that their first months on the job are spent actually learning the beauty trade and unlearning bad habits taught in the beauty school. Again these are generalizations garnered from interviews and do not apply to large "professional" schools, but the elements of mismanagement, lack of professionalism, and very inadequate training seem to be more prevalent than success stories.

But finally the day comes when, having passed the state examination, the young beautician is ready for her first job. She is the fledgling and probably will be fleeced. She has to learn how to get and keep customers; how to get along with her coworkers and boss; how to have customers request her by name—in short, how to survive. One beautician remembered her first job.

It's really hard. You sit on your behind day after day and only help out with shampoos. It's only when someone is really busy or when the weekend comes that you have some customers. You are getting frantic because you have to pay for your chair and you are working on a small salary with the hope of a percentage take—and by damn you don't have any customers. Then you start in finagling and fudging. You can get in good with the receptionist by taking over for her when she wants to go for coffee. That way you can answer the phone and start booking yourself.

Other hairdressers told how they "bad-mouthed" other salons or other beauticians. But that's a dangerous game. If you start to undercut beauticians in the same shop, vendettas can become quite bitter. And the new kid in the salon always loses the battle. More than likely, hairdressers build up a steady clientele based on other beauticians' leftovers. It's a slow process and may involve a whole series of "freebies." One way to get customers is to do hair styling for local charity fashion shows. Not only is the stylist's name on the program, but many women who are volunteer models may come to the shop to have their hair done. Thus, little by little, the hairdresser garners more customers. Hopefully it is a pleasant client-customer relationship, but not always.

Undoubtedly for most women their weekly hair appointment is a simple business transaction. They go to the hairdresser, have their hair shampooed, set, dried, and styled. They pay their bill, tip the beautician, and go home or back to the office. Yet, our interviews with hairdressers in small towns and metropolitan cities show there *is* a darker side.

I conducted a series of interviews which indicated that, like the sadistic husband with a masochistic wife, the gambler and his bookie, or the alcoholic and his favorite bartender, both hairdresser and patron cannot do without each other, yet each despises the other. The hairdresser needs the patron's money and the client the beautician's skill. In order to earn her salary and a tip, the beautician often has to withstand untold abuse but wreaks fearsome vengeance on her customer.

Conflict between patron and beautician arises because the hairdresser is intrinsic to the middle-class milieu but not part of it. The hairdresser is a confidante but not a friend. She listens to cocktail party gossip but never gets invited; she is always the outsider looking in. As a servant, she is treated with the same kind of candor that milady had with the upstairs maid. Like the upstairs maid, the beautician has learned that she should work efficiently and be a toady. Like all Uncle Toms and Uriah Heeps, she must develop strange ways of maintaining her own personal integrity. The giggling beautician passing on stories about a community pillar's tippling and the stony-faced hairdresser calmly chopping her client's hair to shreds are sisters to Malcolm X, who, when he worked in a restaurant in Harlem, used to spit in the dishes of ribs ordered by slumming whites. Such behavior may be weird, but it is ego strengthening.

Hairdressers need every bit of encouragement they can snatch, for they are constantly assaulted by evidence that they never quite belong. Nearly 90 percent of the hairdressers interviewed came from working-class families, and more than half never completed high school. Beauticians who work with middle- and upper-class patrons cater to women whose mores, norms, and very vocabulary are at first foreign and bewildering. By carefully watching, listening, and imitating the life-style of her customers, a beautician seeks to cast aside her plebeian origins. Insecure, unsure of herself, knowing that her father says "ain't," that her mother schleps around in a dirty housecoat, that her brother stabs his meat with his fork, and that her husband punches a time clock, the beautician is pathetically grateful for her momentary association with witty, brittle, facile representatives of the cocktail party set. And she becomes a skilled sycophant.

One of the first things that a hairdresser learns is that women come to beauty salons not only to be stylish but also to fill up empty hours and seek reassurance. Lonely women use the beauty salon as a substitute for the confessional or psychiatrist's couch. Hairdressers are rarely surprised when a customer begins to reveal her psyche on the first visit.

It's incredible. Customer after customer comes in and sits down and then—boom! You start to shampoo her and the first thing you know she is telling you about her sex life, her kids, her husband, God only knows what else. It's scary. I thought maybe there was something about me that caused customers to spill their guts but other girls tell me that the same thing happens to them.

(Thirty-nine-Year-Old Female)

Some hairdressers say that customers are open and free in their confidence because of the indulgent, sybaritic atmosphere of the beauty shop where customers are pampered, spoiled, caressed, and coddled. Beauticians earn large tips for supplying that ''little extra bit'' such as massaging the customer's neck during a shampoo, bringing the patron coffee or magazines while she is under the dryer, brushing imaginary lint from the patron's dress, and constantly reassuring the customer how lovely she is. But their most important function is that of sympathetic listener.

And listen they do. Time and time again hairdressers mentioned that they act like therapists and admitted that they are frightened by their patrons' intimacy. What is even more astounding is that some beauticians reported that their patrons are so upset and so anxious for an attentive ear that they call beauticians at home and, while fortified with bourbon or pills, pour out their troubles to confused and surprised hairdressers.

Yet these ladies who so earnestly unburden themselves do not think of their beautician as a friend. Sadly the hairdresser admits that she is a paid listener. She knows that this is part of her role. She learned in beauty school not to disagree with the customer, not to offer advice, not to volunteer any opinions—in short, never to express herself.

Just as milady of yesteryear whispered her deepest secrets to the upstairs maid and then issued commands in a stentorian tone, so also does today's matron feel it her prerogative to bully and boss her servant-hairdresser. As for the latter, the name of the game is pleasing the customer, but sometimes it can be a vicious game, as one hairdresser angrily expounded:

> I have to make every wrinkled hag in this town look like she's about twenty years old. When I don't get the job done, they sit there and complain like crazy. When I charge fifty cents for a cream rinse, the customer will scream and accuse me of robbing her. But then she comes to me and brags how she paid twenty dollars for a set on her cruise to Bermuda. We make a living by taking other people's abuse. We get treated like dogs. We get shoved around and have to take a lot of non-sense. The customer comes in and is mad about some-thing and takes it out on the girl. I tell you there are days when all the money in the world isn't enough to pay for what I have to take. There are times when my stomach gets tied up in knots.
>
> *(Thirty-eight-Year-Old Female)*

Tension runs high and cannot be relieved just by pounding or kicking a wall. The upstairs maid retaliated by burning madam's best petticoat or lacing her stays too tightly, while present-day beauticians are much more subtle and devious. All beauticians interviewed admitted that they have paid back in malicious kind for real or imagined slights. Every stylist confessed to having deliberately sabotaged a customer. Some have cut a customer's hair so badly that it took months for the hair to grow back in evenly. Others told of being so angry over a customer's having tinted her own hair at home that they added permanent-wave solution to the rinse water, thus stripping the client's hair of the home-applied tint. Conversely, when a patron gave herself a permanent wave at home or, worse, had it done at another shop, then the beautician added neutralizer to the rinse water and ruined the curl. Intentionally hacking, burning, bleaching, and stripping their patrons' hair, beauticians unleash a whole flood of hostilities.

However, most hairdressers, both male and female, agreed that male hairdressers do not suffer the same insult and injury as do women beauticians. Why?

The answer is relatively uncomplicated. Since males in our society receive more deference than females, female patrons are more courteous and less demanding toward male stylists than female beauticians. One hairdresser exploded:

> Hell! All Franco's customers are in love with him. He can't do hair worth a damn but he mutters in their ear and tells them how beautiful they are and they all go ape.
>
> *(Thirty-two-Year-Old Female)*

Of the some twenty male hairdressers interviewed, all agreed that they treated their customers firmly and thus were in control of the patron-customer relationship at all times. They boasted that they didn't hear as much gossip as the girls because when things got too intimate, they (the men) immediately changed the subject. But deference is hardly a quality in male hairdressers. One of my favorite male hairdressers used to snarl at his customers. Another would hit a misbehaving customer on the head with a hairbrush and tell her to "straighten up and behave!" Female customers seem to adore their male hairdressers.

How "male" are the "male" hairdressers? Are all male stylists "gay"? Who knows? Since we don't know the true percentage of homosexuals in the population as a whole, there is no reason to assume that male hairdressers have a greater or lesser preponderance of gay men. In both professional and personal dealings with male hairdressers, I found their sexual preference running from wild, amoral heterosexuality to dull, happily married family man to flaming gay. Some male hairdressers are admittedly bisexual. To what degree I don't know. It may be that the traditionally stereotypical "gay occupations," such as hairdresser, interior decorator, and ballet dancer, do indeed attract and contain a larger percentage of male homosexuals than the general population. However it may be just as likely that these occupations have demonstrated a sympathetic or at least tolerant attitude toward gay males and thus the male homosexual does not have to hide his sexual preference. That is, we have no idea how many male homosexual lawyers or doctors there are, but we are pretty safe in assuming that these professions do not tolerate sexual ambiguity to any degree and the gay doctor or lawyer has indeed to be a closet or weekend homosexual.

Nonetheless we should note that, even though almost 90 percent of beauticians are women, wealth and power are concentrated in the hands of men. More men are shop owners, school owners, product demonstrators, and important members of state and national cosmetologist associations than are women. Female colleagues as well as female customers defer to male hairdressers. Or are men more ambitious and harder-working than women? That's what all the male and some female beauticians said. However, remember that we are referring to a woman's occupation with all the attendant problems of femaleness. Even though times are changin', career commitment is not necessarily a feminine characteristic. Nursing, library science, grade-school teaching, and hairdressing are "in and out" professions. That is, women work after finishing school, drop out to marry and have a family, come to work part-time when the children are small, and return full-time when the children are in high school or when divorce or death hits. Again, this is the usual sporadic female work-pattern, but it has drastically changed with the advent of the pill (and spacing or complete prevention of pregnancy) and because of an often desperate need for a second income. But of those women who are full-time beauticians, few are shop owners and fewer still big-time hair stylists and school owners.

There is a chicken-egg analysis at work here too. Maybe women are indeed just as career committed as men, but women have trouble getting financing from banks, have no established credit lines, and usually do not get management experience in their early working years. Some women beauticians complain bitterly that there is a closed homosexual conspiracy in the "big time." That is, gay men promote their gay protégés on the convention/stylist/show/ competition circuit. That may be so, but it seems to be inadequate explanation. Perhaps more important, men are motivated to make big money quickly. Women have the

wish but not the drive. And that's purely and simply sociali-
zation. Blatant discrimination against women—whether by
bank loan officers or gay hairdressers—does not tell you
why so many leaders in the hairdresser-cosmetologist industry are men. Women are socialized to think that they
cannot get ahead, are inferior, will fail, and it isn't ladylike
to hustle with the guys. Men are told to be aggressive, get
ahead, succeed, and undercut the other fellow.

So that's a partial explanation of why men are more
successful than women in the world of business in general
and the beauty business in particular. But the male-female
sex game is still alive and well here too. That is, women do
defer, coo, and flutter around a man (even a gay man), and
many women express preference for a male hairdresser. If
you accept the fact that a woman is getting her hair done to
be personally attractive, neat, and sexually interesting, then
it stands to reason that a male stylist should do a "better"
job than a woman—a man knows what other men like. Or
some silly reasoning like that. Strange subordinate-superior
client-patron relationships develop. As we noted previously, women customers mind their p's and q's with male
hairdressers.

But the ambience of the shop is as important a variable
as the sex of the beautician in explaining the intensity of
customer-patron warfare. As we shall see, there is a basic
typology of beauty shops with corresponding different
modes of patron-customer behavior in each.

First of all, there is the *boiler factory*. The boiler
factory is reminiscent of most tawdry, overcrowded beauty
colleges. Beauticians range on each side of a long, narrow,

rather dingy room. Hairdressers are often young graduates, quite inexperienced, and more often than not foreign nationals (Chinese, Latin American, Iranian, and maybe Greek). These girls hardly speak English, provide their own curlers, brushes, and combs, and buy supplies from the shop owner. The money-making scheme of beauty school is repeated here once again. Owners buy supplies at huge discounts and resell them to the girls at a decided markup— even though still under the beautician's regular discount price. Like beauty-school customers, boiler-factory customers obtain a bargain and a rip-off. That is, they get an inexpensive hairdo or permanent from an inexperienced beautician. Sometimes you find an undiscovered gem in the boiler factory—a competent and imaginative stylist. Mostly, though, the girls are inexperienced and harried. Volume is the secret of boiler-factory hairdressing. Advertisements emphasize that there is no waiting, no appointment necessary, and cut-rate prices to boot. Speed is of the essence. Beauticians who cannot handle a rapid and constant turnover of customers are fired. Boiler factories keep long hours. Some are open from seven in the morning (to get the early-bird crowd) to seven or eight at night (to get the after-work bunch). Some boiler factories are open on Sundays and others stay open until two or three o'clock in the morning. I often wondered what kind of person got her hair done in the wee hours of the morning and so I went to a couple of these establishments to find out. Suffice it to say that the hennaed/bleached white-plastic-booted clientele confirmed my suspicions. At midnight, in one shop, a fresh-faced brownette with streaks of blond in her long, flowing locks argued furiously with the manager. This sweet young thing with a faint midwestern accent who looked like everybody's kid sister from Iowa was accompanied by a swinging black dude in a white suit. The girl was desperately trying to wheedle her own way.

> Look, I'll pay *anything* or *do* anything to get my hair streaked for tonight. I've got my main man here and he's made some whole lot of arrangements for me. I can't go around with stringy hair and dark roots. He won't let me. Now, I've been coming here for a long time and you've always treated me good. This time it's an emergency. My whole career is at stake.

Career! One look at the black dude lounging against the appointment desk and a hurried conversation in Spanish followed between the operators and the owner. Given the striking emergency—the pantherlike dude and a career at stake—one of the girls agreed to work overtime. But boiler factories are designed for quick/fast/rapid turnover and cater to everyone and anyone. You pays your two dollars and you gets your hairdo. No fuss. No nonsense. And if you're lucky some style.

Style is unimportant in the next kind of shop—the *mom 'n pop shop.* This is the neighborhood beauty parlor most often located in the back part of a house, a basement, or a small renovated store. There is usually only one owner-manager-operator, or sometimes on weekends another girl helps out. Styles come and go infrequently in this shop, hairdos lagging some five years behind the current fad; still the shop stays in business because the overweight clients know that even though they can never be beautiful, they can get a neat hairdo that doesn't "fall out." The clientele all know one another, usually live within walking distance of the shop, and are most often working-class wives who cannot afford downtown prices. Because patrons and beautician are from the same social class and often in the same age range, conflict is at a minimum. The shop has a cozy, homy atmosphere redolent with the smell of freshly baked brownies brought by one of the patrons.

I have had great fun in mom 'n pop shops throughout the United States and in other tucked-away spots in Europe and Latin America. One of the major occupations of the mom 'n pop shop is gossip. If you want to find out who is sleeping with whom, who is getting or contemplating a divorce, who has had a serious operation, or what local political scandals abound—go to your local mom 'n pop shop. Gossip is not too widespread a commodity in the boiler factory or in soigné shops. In the boiler factory the turnover rate of customers is so high that one customer isn't interested in another, so gossip must be concentrated on the Elizabeth Taylor-Jackie Onassis level. In the soigné upper-class shop (as we shall see later), gossip is death because the customers know each other only too well. But gossip is life itself to the mom 'n pop'ers.

I have stood outside my neighborhood shop in Buenos Aires and gossiped with the clientele as to what general's wife was getting her hair done more frequently than usual and thus gained some insight into the cocktail party circuit of Buenos Aires and the lives of the military in a *coup* situation. In my favorite mom 'n pop shop in West Virginia I found out about the local moonshiners, tourist peccadilloes, and how to make the best apple butter ever. Another mom 'n pop shop near Chicago that I patronized kept me breathlessly informed as to a local millionaire's penchant for wife beating. Still another in Maryland is better than a rest cure. Whenever I appear in desperation, seeking instant wash and set, the manager coos and clucks over my rush, tells me how brilliant and beautiful I am, serves me coffee and cookies, admires my clothes and jewelry, and generally boosts my morale to such an extreme that I am soothed and surfeited with loving ego strokes.

As much as customers like mom 'n pop shops, other hairdressers dislike the mom 'n pop'ers with a vengeance. The reason is financial. Given that the mom 'n pop shops are located in a home or in a renovated garage, there is little or no overhead and thus prices can be cut. The owner buys her supplies at the regular shop-owner discount and can afford to pass the savings on to her customer. Now it is obvious why the shop owner in a high-rent district or even the modest shop owner in a shopping center is incensed by the mom 'n pop'ers. Even the IRS is into the act. Mom 'n pop shops keep slipshod records and often don't total up accounts too well—intentionally or not—when income tax time rolls around. Even Ma Bell has to check regularly on the mom 'n pop'ers. Often the mom 'n pop shop simply has a residence telephone, and only after Ma Bell runs a check or receives a complaint does the mom 'n pop proprietor pay for a business telephone.

Their peccadilloes are many but the mom 'n pop'ers still predominate in mostly lower-middle and working-class districts. They cater to neighbors and friends, and business is easy and nonrushed. It's only when the shop becomes successful that the atmosphere is destroyed. The owner hires a shampoo girl, then hires another beautician, customers begin to demand more style, new techniques are introduced, and suddenly it is a real honest-to-God beauty salon and not a neighborhood kaffee-klatch-cum-girls'-dormitory.

But the next kind of shop still has fun overtones at least, and that's why we call it the *play shop*. In the play shop, operators have more fun than the patrons. Usually the beauticians are young, single girls in their late teens or early twenties who worry more about boyfriends, dates, pending engagements, and silver patterns than they do about customer satisfaction. Giggling and chattering endlessly to each other over their patrons' heads, the girls address a few comments to the customers but focus their attention on their fellow beauticians. These hairdressers spend most of their workday experimenting on each other and are constantly seen wearing rollers so that they can be prepared for the evening's date. In some shops, play is the essence of the day. Silly practical jokes go on all the time: hiding supplies, switching lunch orders, pretending that one of the girls received a ratty wig. Giggles and high-pitched squeals punctuate ringing telephones and whirring dryers. Some play shops regularly plan parties around significant holidays: Christmas, Valentine's Day, St. Patrick's Day.

One shop I used to patronize had a regular dress-up costume fiesta for Halloween. The operators came dressed as Raggedy Ann or space pilots or Wolf Man. Their ingenuity and creativity matched any costume party ball or carnival dress I have ever seen.

These play-shop antics contribute to a sense of belonging or group solidarity, but contribute nothing to professionalism. Since the operators are usually young, play-shop owners use these mad methods in an attempt to keep their girls amused so that operators will stay with the shop and not drift away. Operators make valiant attempts to approximate high-fashion style. They usually don't succeed because the operators don't have the time or money to attend styling school or major conventions. But the play shop giggles on. Things would be so much better for the beauticians if they could experiment only on each other and not be bothered by customers.

Customers are young, white-collar, married women who want more style than can be found in mom 'n pop shops but who also cannot afford chic salon prices. Unfortunately, they cannot afford baby-sitters either and bring their bored, cranky children to the shop. Patrons become increasingly annoyed at the beauticians' antics, while operators are irritated by their patrons' undisciplined children roaming through the shop. Each patron wants her beautician's undivided attention, while the hairdresser wishes that the customer would leave and take her brat with her. Both patron and customer snap at each other. The hairdresser yanks her customer's hair, or turns the dryer to its highest setting, or uses any of a hundred tricks to bedevil and harass the customer.

Needless to say, the play shop has a heavy turnover of customers. The beauticians also come and go, aimlessly drifting into marriage and out of hairdressing.

While the play shop is a madhouse of children and hee-hawing beauticians, the *mod shop* is a noisy, bustling maelstrom, where customers and beauticians run about in manic confusion. Hard acid rock blares from stereo speakers hung around the walls; whirling colored lights reflect an insane pattern on the chrome and glass fixtures; operators are young males who lisp and wear the ultimate in fashion; patrons smoke furiously and tap their watches nervously because their favorite operator is always running a half-hour off schedule.

Customers are young, lower-middle-class models, secretaries, and students who want to be *au courant* in order to be as attractive as possible to whatever young man on the rise (or old man already risen) would like to support them. Beauty is a necessary commodity for the patron's success. No wonder then that temper tantrums are the medium of communication.

In the mod shop the majority of stylists are male. Note they are called "stylist," never hairdresser, and God forbid that you should say "beautician" or "operator." And male stylists are able to dominate the situation. Periodically one of the stylists will have a violent argument with one of his customers, throw down his comb and scissors in a pout, and stomp out of the shop, leaving a surprised woman with her hair half shorn. Usually, however, there is a mutual admiration between customer and stylist—the stylist assuring the patron that she is a model of up-to-date fashion and the customer crooning that her modish look is due solely to his skill.

Skill and talent he has. The mod shop and the mod stylist can parlay *chutzpah* flattery and some ingenuity to small or large fortunes. Vidal Sassoon is a case in point. With skill and flair he has become a multimillionaire whose styles are repeated and copied throughout the world. On somewhat smaller scales are chic stylists in large cities who are quoted and interviewed on television and in newspaper women's style sections. These men too are, if not millionaires, damn close to it. Chains of mod boutique salons develop. These prominent stylists proclaim their message regarding cut, style, and shape on the pages of *Vogue* and even *Time* and *Newsweek.* The beehive is out. Migod, it is really out and only seen on the heads of country western singers. The shag is gone. The wedge is in. And of course, soon the wedge will be out and probably we will be piling wigs and hairpieces on top of our heads like so many more Marie Antoinettes. Looking good is not the issue for patron and stylist in the mod shop—looking *in* is important.

A current wave in mod shops is the unisex shop, with unisex cuts and I am sure unisexual or bisexual stylists. Music pounds through speakers, walls are usually covered in metallic aluminum sheeting, and sheer madness prevails. Customers are indeed unisex, for it is hard to tell who is who or what in blue jeans and field jackets. Lately, western leisure suits with flowered blouse shirts are the current rage.

Dutch-boy bobs are in and teasing is out. The frantic mod-shop atmosphere repeats the tension of a dating bar. Everyone is convinced that she is going to have a good time but no one does. In the mod shop everyone is convinced that she is chic and worldly and yet most are smothered in insecurities. And the beat goes on.

In deliberate and studied contrast to clamorous shops of the hoi polloi, the most distinctive feature of the *snob shop* is its studied and restive silence. The snob shop caters to the "carriage trade" and its upper-upper-class customers never bring their children to the shop. As a matter of fact, the customers rarely see their children, whom they pop into boarding school as early as possible. As for the reference to "carriage trade," the snob shop indeed is the last outpost of the chauffeured limousine—with or without diplomatic plates. This of course does not imply that the snob shop caters only to elderly grande dames and portly matrons—albeit those do comprise the majority of customers—but rather to the Main Line, Gold Coast, Grosse Pointe crowd in cashmere sweaters with quiet strand of pearls. The horsey set. The "don't-I-remember-you-from-boarding-school-in-Lausanne?" set. The "aren't-emeralds-so-very-vulgar?" set. The secure old-moneyed and long-standing aristocracy set. With a few exceptions, of course.

Catering to the snob shop clientele is not easy. Ladies of leisure and breeding don't want to go to mod shops and in actuality for big occasions have the hair stylist *come* to their own boudoir. But for those who do actually set foot in a hair salon—the salon must be comparable to one's own comfortable living quarters. Usually the snob shop is owned and managed by an aging homosexual who has devoted many hours to the subtle but elegant decor of crystal chandeliers, Wedgwood bowls, and assorted chinoiserie. Patrons change out of their designer clothes upon arriving at the shop and sit under the dryer in pink, blue, or flowered smocks. Patrons sip coffee out of white china cups with a delicate gold rim—paper and plastic are awfully vulgar, you know. Indeed the coffeepot is hidden in the back room away from sight and sound of customers. Gossip is rare in the snob shop. Actually gossip is prohibited. Customers are important people and/or wives of important people. The least bit or whiff of scandal repeated under the dryer or passed on by a bitchy hair stylist could cause irreparable harm. No gossip. No, thank you. That is not to say that the customers themselves do not engage in a little character assassination here and there but all with the subtlety of a stiletto. The major concern in the snob shop is to have one's hair styled—but not too high style—and to move on to luncheon, fashion show, charity bazaar, gym class, or whatever.

These patrons too are seeking the elusive Grail of Beauty, and become annoyed when they don't attain it. Stylists in these shops carefully guard their tempers, knowing that bountiful tips and Christmas checks depend on their being ingratiating. Hairdressers who have worked in various types of salons told me that customers in snob shops are the least courteous. However, it should be noted that there is a variation in gentility and good manners, because hairdressers report that nouveau riche super-upwardly mobile and status-marginal women inflict greater verbal abuse on their hairdressers than do socially secure upper-uppers. A nouvelle arrivée, the upwardly mobile woman, is understandably nervous and correspondingly nasty. Ms. Nouveau Riche comes to the most chic salon in the city to associate with the "in" group, receive the unctuous care of the stylist, acquire the current mode look, and thus peripherally belong. In turn, the stylist, sensing her nervousness and knowing that she is not to the purple born, may play all sorts of malevolent tricks on the unsuspecting patron, or indeed deliberately misstyle the customer's hair, all the while assuring her that it is flattering, as quid pro quo for the patron's bad manners.

Why do beautician and customer tolerate this strange symbiotic love-hate relationship of scorn alternating with adoration that seems to be a feature of every beauty salon? It is far too facile to explain the seething undercurrents in beauty salons in terms of customer neuroticism, status differences, or the upstairs-maid syndrome, although these are reasonable enough explanations in themselves. For it matters not whether the shop is decorated in early bordello or late Howard Johnson's, patronized by long, leggy models or lumpy, fortyish matrons; everyone gets some sort of ego boost and tension release.

Some customers enjoy shredding their psyche into bits, while others like to listen to patrons bellow at each other over the whir of dryers and the sad tales of teen-age drug abuse and assorted marital problems, and still others find satisfaction in bullying the beautician. Hairdressers find satisfaction in serving the great, near-great, rich, and near-rich, or waging a personal vendetta against anyone who attacks the beautician's integrity in any way.

But rich or poor, teeny-bopper or pensioner, neurotic or near-normal, all—the hairdressers and the customers—are caught in the beauty trap. Not one beautician in the sample ever questioned the morality or value of "looking nice," because hairdressers earn their salaries by selling dreams and assuring every Plain Jane that she will be transformed into Raquel Welch. Hairdresser and client know that "looking nice" is a prime virtue in American society, for beauty is the lure in which women trap their men, keep their men, entice their men, and attain financial security. Beautician and patron firmly believe that a new hair style will calm inner tensions, help a flagging marriage, and boost morale.

Both are victims lured by Narcissus' siren call. Hairdresser and customer are linked together in an unholy alliance of cutting, slashing, burning, waving, and bleaching. The customer who wheedles and coaxes for an appointment turns mean when her same tired face stares at her from the mirror after several hours of the stylist's care. Frantically attending their petulant charges, stylists suffer nasty customers, sore feet, varicose veins, cracked and bleeding hands, and frayed tempers. This is the beauty trap. This is why beautician and client are forever locked in mortal combat. The surprise is not that the hairdresser is unable to perform her fairy godmother tricks but that beautician and customer unequivocally believe that it can be done. The sorrow is that so many are in need of such magic.

And they sit under the dryer immersed in what is

going-to-be. Some of them peek at pulpy passion magazines and others devour ads and articles in *Vogue* or *Harper's* dealing with what is the "in" color for lipstick or the current cosmetic surgery discovery. A new dream from a jar or a realized transformation courtesy of Blue Cross and the surgeon's scalpel. Painting and pasting, cutting and trimming. That's the next saga.

5 Paint. Paste. and Cut

Kohl, henna, rouge, rice powder, paint pots—from cave-women through Egyptian queens, medieval princesses, and my pristine grandmother, painting and primping, crimping and curling have been part of the feminine way of life. Cosmetics for women (and sometimes men) are part of human tradition and condition. In the United States the cosmetics industry is worth nearly $7 billion per year. Indeed the first black millionaire, who also happened to be female and thus the first black and/or woman millionaire, was a Madame Walker, who answered the need for black women to have their own cosmetics attuned to black skin tones and skin types. The cosmetic industry has, as is well known, been the forte of many women—Elizabeth Arden,

Madame Rubinstein, and the local Avon lady who earns money by ringing other women's doorbells.

With enough advertising and puffed hype, any product can be merchandised—but cosmetics all the more easily. Compare the array of cosmetics on any woman's dressing table or medicine cabinet shelves with the paltry few creams of my grandmother's day and you see how the business has grown and prospered. A need can be created and a product manufactured to answer the huckstered need. All you have to do is to tell women that they *need* shiny bright red lipstick or feminine douches and they will decide—amazingly enough—that they really do *need* a hitherto unknown and unproduced product. Feminine douches are a case in point.

Some five years ago most douches were antiseptic solutions hidden in the back of the medicine closet. Jerry Della Femina, who named the douche Feminique after himself with puckish perverse wit, helped to tout the joys of feminine douches. Douches suddenly appeared in all new varieties of flavors and scents. No doubt the sexual significance of new scents and flavors was somehow related to sexual liberation and the delights of oral sex. Nevertheless, young and old, liberated or inhibited, more and more women bought feminine douches. The problem was—and is— that douches are cosmetics and not patent medicines. If douches were considered to be patent medicines—like aspirin or a poison ivy remedy—then their regulation would be more stringent. More's the pity. More's the pity for thousands of women who have suffered adverse reactions such as burning of genitals, painful inflammation, and even extended hospital stays—courtesy of the feminine douche/spray fad. Where is there social responsibility on the part of the cosmetics industry or the advertising agencies who thought up one more travesty of advertising? Create the need. Fill the need. Charge an exorbitant price for fulfilling the need. And the buyer be damned.

It is distressing to realize that most lipsticks contain 3 to 10 cents' worth of ingredients and sell for anywhere from $1 to $3. Now that kind of profit may be regarded as somewhat extravagant. Even cold cream, with about 50 cents in ingredients, ranges from $2 to $6. When a manufacturer claims exotic ingredients for a cold cream—for example, secretions from the queen bee—then the sky's the limit, or at least $50 for a few ounces. Venal manufacturers realize that wild, exaggerated advertising will lure gullible customers. Because laws governing cosmetics are so lax, the public is duped again. Neither the FDA in particular nor the public in general understands the effect the some four thousand chemicals used in the manufacture of cosmetics may have. But the National Commission on Product Safety estimates that as many as sixty thousand people or more are injured by cosmetics *each year* and that thirty million Americans are allergy prone.

Horror piles upon horror. Skin infections. Blindness. Loss of hair. The kind of horror story that no one wants to hear. Sometimes there is a back-to-nature kind of feature in one of the women's magazines stating that natural food products will do just as well as—if not better than—most cosmetics. Use mayonnaise to soften your hands. Warm up olive oil and pour it over your hair to correct dry frizzy hair. Use a masque of crushed avocados to soften the face. It's fun for a while, even though messy. But the soft glowing lights of the department-store cosmetics counter are so much more alluring than one's refrigerator.

For those convinced that they have allergy-prone skins, only two companies, Almay of New York and Ar-Ex of Chicago, publish lists of the ingredients omitted from their products, and along with some other companies, will freely disclose what *is* in their products if asked. After years of delaying tactics by the cosmetics manufacturers, a new regulation will soon go into effect requiring all companies to list the contents of their products on package labels. You have to translate the language on the labels, of course, but it's a step in the right direction. Still, there's nothing that prevents a manufacturer from putting anything he wants in a cosmetic. Even if the product is called "hypo-allergenic," that doesn't mean a diddly-damn because it doesn't guarantee it is hypo-allergenic for *you.* The loose legislation governing safe and pure cosmetics is nonsense. Some poor creature with a skin allergy can still pay a high price for a shoddy product and have her skin break out. It's not that the consumer is ignorant or stupid but only that we are ready to believe the printed word. If a product says hypo-allergenic, then, assuming government protection and consumer advocacy in Congress, we assume that is what the product really is. Not so. There is some hope, however; whispers are heard in the halls of Congress and to a teeny extent in the cosmetics-company laboratories that the consumer needs some *bona fide* guarantees. What will probably be necessary to achieve this protection is a plague of constant and ever increasing law suits from dissatisfied and wounded customers. When the cosmetics industry finds out that it stands to lose thousands upon thousands of dollars, then it will police itself. And only then.

While a wholesale denunciation of the cosmetics industry is perhaps unduly harsh, so also is an indictment of cosmetic surgeons. Cosmetic surgery has a justifiable place in the medical specialties. A woman with severe facial burns restored. Children with hare lips and cleft palates made normal. A young man with scars from an automobile accident made whole once again. Men and women having disfiguring birthmarks suddenly obliterated. These are success stories of cosmetic surgery. Do new noses, face lifts, silicone implants, and buttock reductions contribute to psychological well-being? The answer is both yes and no.

Magical transformations abound in children's literature: dirty scullery maid into princess; nasty long-nosed puppet into charming little boy; and slimy frog into prince. Although we are assured that our favorite characters lived-happily-ever-after, in all likelihood they suffered some acute psychological trauma. Maybe Cinderella exhibited dreadful table manners at royal banquets. Perhaps Pinocchio awoke in terror every night thinking that his nose had grown longer. Possibly the prince wanted to wallow once again in his stagnant frog pond. This ambivalence explains problems between cosmetic surgeons and their patients. One surgeon whom I interviewed told me about the surgeon's constant fears of a malpractice suit.

The cosmetic surgeon is the one surgeon who gets sued over and over again.

You are dealing with highly upset and pretty damned weird people! A woman who thinks that an eyelid lift and removing a few wrinkles will gloriously change her life for the better is betting on the wrong horse. I try and avoid those types but every once in a while I'm wrong. That's not to say that there aren't people who are unhappy with the way they look. As a matter of fact, they ought to be unhappy because they some- times look like hell! A stitch here and a sew there and they won't win any beauty contests but will no longer be freaks. That's my kind of patient. Imagine what it's like to be called "Dumbo" for years because your ears stick out worse than Clark Gable's. Then along comes the magic wonder of surgery and the ears don't stick out anymore. I've had a teen-age boy sit and cry his heart out with joy after the bandages were taken off and his ears didn't stick out.

Why did the other kids call the boy "Dumbo"? Why does a flat-chested woman cry herself to sleep night after night? Why do teen-agers seek contact lenses? Why do parents spend thousands and thousands of dollars on or- thodontia that may be for cosmetic purposes only? Obvi- ously to meet the standards of beauty of our society. Beauty is ephemeral but can be defined. The "California look" epitomizes what U.S. beauty standards are all about. The California man or woman is tanned of limb, straight of teeth, short of nose, blond of hair, and without a spare ounce of fat. The man has rippling muscles and the woman soft-rounded contours with big round breasts. No wonder then that at puberty Jewish boys get Bar-Mitzvahed and Jewish girls get new noses. The hair-dye industry flourishes and the cosmetic surgeon wields his expensive magic scalpel with the aplomb of a medieval sorcerer. Patients seek out a cosmetic surgeon because more nonsense than sense appears in popular magazines extolling the virtues of the ''latest'' surgery techniques. It is very difficult to find out exact statistics on cosmetic surgery because sometimes these procedures are disguised as noncosmetic so that the patient can collect from the insurance company. Medical journals also only cautiously explore new procedures. Unfortunately medical journals also use only small samples and rather incomplete descriptions. There is very little popular literature describing the ''ifs-and-buts'' of cosmetic surgery.[3] Patients trust that cosmetic surgeons are magicians.

Yet this magic is not always effective. Most cosmetic surgeons are competent. Some are not. The ravages of the incompetent are borne by their willing victims. Some women who sought to have wrinkles removed from their face now wear permanent grimaces because facial nerves were severed. Surgeons who promise to remove acne scars sometimes remove part of the face as well. The vagaries and dangers of silicone implantation are well enough known.

All surgery is dangerous, even if it is ''simple'' surgery like an appendix operation. However most surgery does not have to be repeated. But wrinkles do come back. Fat does reappear on thighs and buttocks. And the operations are repeated. Further, most women are apparently unaware of the deep heavy scarring that occurs after a thigh or buttock-lift operation. The fat is gone, the skin is tightened, but the patient has a crisscross patchwork of scars that may or may not lighten *in a few years.*

Cosmetic surgery is a direct outgrowth of Madison Avenue mass-media mush in combination with the Protestant ethic. The patient seems to think that if he/she suffers under the knife, pays a goodly sum to a surgeon, endures postoperative trauma and pain, then he/she will deserve the gift of beauty. Suffer and you shall be rewarded. The reward is the approbation of the world. Just 'tain't so. One surgeon explains:

> I thought in medical school that they were handing us a bunch of bull about the patient who goes shopping for surgery. I'm talking about the woman who comes into your office with a picture of Elizabeth Taylor and says that she wants Elizabeth Taylor's face. Jesus! I just say I can't do it but refer her to this son-of-a-bitch I know who specializes in Elizabeth Taylor faces. Or there's the other kind, who walks in with a picture of a nose. Just the nose. She probably yanked it out of some photograph in *Vogue* magazine. That's the nose she wants. I'm just some kind of errand boy who will give her this wonderful nose. Of course that doesn't take into consideration bone structure, cartilage, and the anatomy of *her* face. That lady worries me! She'll see me in court because she didn't get the nose she wanted. They never get the noses they want, those broadies. Right? Or the other lulu is the one who comes to you

with the story about how she has had three nose jobs. None of them were any good. She wants me to do the fourth nose job. No way. She also is going to take me to court like she took those three other suckers before me.

Notice that the doctor refers to his patients as "she." Of course. Women patients outnumber men no matter what the specialty—including urology. Cosmetic surgeons estimate that their practices are 60 percent female. The clientele of some doctors is exclusively female—that is, those who specialize in fat reduction: tightening thighs, removing blubber from buttocks, and removing folds of fat from stomachs. Women patients seek cosmetic surgery because women are more beauty conscious than men. Interestingly, though, cosmetic surgeons report that lately more and more men are coming to them for face lifts. The youth-beauty culture fetish has hit the aging executive. Wrinkles and sagging jowls are no longer the hallmark of a successful and well-seasoned veteran but simply of someone over the hill; marks of someone who may no longer be needed in the board room. So men are buying the message that health-beauty-youth add up to success. Witness Senator Proxmire's hair transplant.

Yet the surgeons whom I interviewed all begged to remain anonymous. None would allow his name to be used as a reference. They were all afraid of meeting me again one day in court. It was a reasonable fear because the cosmetic surgeon has always been sued with greater frequency than other doctors. However, with the current proliferation of malpractice suits in all specialties, the cosmetic surgeon is losing his lead in the courtroom game. More than anything else, though, the surgeons themselves were hard pressed to justify their own existence. Some didn't give a damn, like this doctor:

> I am in this business to make money. Just like a dermatologist or an ophthalmologist, I make money. Lots and lots of money. Nose jobs and face lifts are fine with me because they pay for my mortgage and my vacations in the Caribbean. I never had any illusions about saving lives or fighting beri-beri in some god-forsaken jungle. I wanted to be a money-grubbing son-of-a-bitch with three big cars. And I am.

While this surgeon's honesty is surprising and fits a stereotypical image of the high-priced society surgeon, he may be too defensive. Cosmetic surgeons who specialize in ''beauty'' answer a need. It is a psychic need. Maybe a neurotic need. Such surgery may indeed save a life—at least the psychological life of an individual. While it seems at first glance that ours is a strange society that has a profession of medical men whose specialty is shortening noses, there is historical and social precedent for the cosmetic surgeon. Ears have been slit and lengthened, noses slit, heads deformed, lips rounded and extended by the local cosmetic surgeon-witch doctor. Since the dawn of time, man has diddled and fiddled around with his (or her) body in order to meet the demands of the local definition of what is or is not lovely, gorgeous, or beautiful.

Anthropologists for years pointed out that the Ubangi women with their huge deformed stretched upper lips were proof that one man's definition of beauty is ugliness to another. We accepted the fact that Ubangi men thought that their plate-billed duck-lipped women were delightful creatures. No one asked the Ubangi. Finally some enterprising young anthropologist asked the Ubangi men what socio-sexual significance these deformations had for the Ubangi tribesmen. The Ubangi replied that their women were the ugliest creatures on the face of the earth. It seems that the Ubangi traditionally were a weak tribe whose neighbors constantly marauded and raided the tribe, carrying off its women. The Ubangi, therefore, deliberately uglified their women so that they would be so unattractive and repulsive that no one would raid or maraud the area again.

Just as the Ubangi had a standard of beauty and counteracted it, so our cosmetic surgeons use every trick in their bag to assure that members of our tribe will appear beautiful and youthful to each other. So there is a place for the nose bobbers that will survive as long as bank accounts can stretch or insurance policies be twisted. Women will haunt the offices of the cosmetic surgeon anxiously looking for the Elizabeth Taylor face. I wonder if anyone has requested a Barbra Streisand nose?

Probably not. But cosmetic surgeons are not the only doctors in the beauty business. While a cosmetic surgeon works on the exterior, there is a small group of surgeons who are into the weight reduction business via the jejunal bypass. Currently, the sure cure for obesity is the jejunal bypass operation. Called the "shunt" or "bypass" among the in group, this operation consists of bypassing a large part of the small intestine and connecting the jejunum to the ileum. Bypassing the small intestine shortens the digestive tract, and regardless of how much the patient eats, he will lose weight because calorie absorption is correspondingly reduced. What could be more perfect for the foodaholic than a surgical operation that guarantees weight loss with no change in eating habits? The fattie can still eat his gigantic meals but will become thin and no longer be treated as a freak.

Beware of such sophistry as this! Greek mythology teaches us that the gods never give gifts without exacting payment. In the case of the bypass operation, the payment may be dehydration, mental illness, and perhaps death, for any operation is a surgical risk, whether for tonsils, in-grown toenails, or jejunal bypass. Here is an excerpt from my notes as I observed my first jejunal bypass.

The operating room is extremely cold and several of the nurses are wearing sweaters. I wish I had put one on too. This is my first operation and I'm beginning to regret the fact that I'm here. I begin to get extremely nervous and wonder if I will make an idiot of myself by fainting.

The surgeons are standing around a huge lump on the table that faintly resembles a cow. I have watched surgery at the university veterinary school and I swear that cows even looked smaller. I'm being ridiculous. It is a human being.

"Well, well, it's Dr. Kinzer," says one of the

green-masked figures. "How are you today? We have reserved a box seat for you." The other residents begin to giggle at this joke because the box seat is precisely that—a box for me to stand on. "Please don't faint forward and for God's sake, don't faint backwards because you'll bitch up the anesthesia equipment. If you think you are going to faint, sit down right away." I think that I'm going to faint now. No, I can't. I asked for it and I'm here.

"O.K., gentlemen, it's cut and paste time," says the head surgeon. They cut and cut. It's the wildest thing. The patient is 469 pounds and cutting through her is like movies I show to my anthropology class of Eskimos cutting whale blubber. I leave and go out for coffee and gossip with the nurses. I come back and the surgeons are still cutting. I leave again for more coffee and when I return they are still cutting and tying. By now I am not afraid of my reactions to the operation but quite bored. Then, there is a flap between the anesthesiologist and the surgeon. There are three anesthesiologists because the tricky part of the operation hinges around the anesthesia. Apparently fat absorbs anesthetics and there is no way to gauge adequately how much anesthetic to give someone who is two to three times normal body weight. The anesthesiologist and his *three* assistants tell the surgeon that he will have to stop for a while, until the patient comes out of this. During the recess, the surgeons change gowns, tell jokes, comment on the sexual availability of the scrub nurse, and generally ignore the patient.

Back to the drawing board, gentlemen. Yukkk. The inside of this woman is incredible. I have seen pictures of operations but this is wild. The intestines are bloated beyond anything I could imagine and are encircled with globs of fat. It's not the blood and guts that bothers me. It's the fat. One of the residents looks up and says to me, "Hey, Doc, ever been on a pig farm? Well, this looks familiar as hell to me." I start to think about how much food a 469-pound woman has to eat. What her life is like. The head surgeon suggests lunch and I accept. I drink black coffee and forgo the lunch.

This procedure is still being performed at this writing in a midwestern medical school. The head surgeon at Midwest was only going to do two or three jejunal bypass operations to give his resident interns some experience. And no more. But he happened to be performing this operation at the time that national publicity popularized Al Hirt's bypass operation. Midwest's public relations department thought it was getting some free publicity for Midwest's Medical Center when it released a story that Dr. James Michaels was also doing the jejunal bypass operation. What a mistake! The day after the newspaper story appeared, the whole Midwest Medical Center switchboard completely burnt out with over *one thousand* calls from people wanting to have the bypass or "fat" operation. Midwest Medical Center was in an uproar because no one could get calls into or out of the medical center—because fatties from as far away as twelve hundred miles were calling to see when they could be scheduled for surgery.

Michaels was overwhelmed at how insistent the callers were. He refused to take any patients unless they were referred by a family physician, were two to three times their normal weight, had no history of liver or heart disease, and many other provisions. And still they came. Rather than making a reputation as a teaching surgeon, he quickly acquired the reputation of being ''the fat surgeon.'' Some of his fellow surgeons referred to Michaels behind his back as ''Midwest's Pitanguy.'' (Pitanguy is a Brazilian surgeon who molds flabby thighs, riding-breeches buttocks, and droopy boobs into firm contours—for an enormous fee, of course.) Michaels' ego was constantly soothed by the adoration and slavering gratitude of his obese patients. With cunning born out of years of rejection, the superobese knew that Michaels was the key to granting them the operation. Before and after the operation, they treated Michaels as some sort of God-on-earth, always referring to him as ''wonderful,'' ''marvelous,'' ''fantastic.''

Almost unwittingly, Michaels became part of the beauty-obesity-magic con game. I don't mean to intimate that Michaels began his career as a fat surgeon. He just seemed to slip and slide into being *the* fat surgeon of one area of the Midwest. More than anything else, his fame spread by word of mouth. One relative told another. A hairdresser would tell a grossly overweight client about a former 300-pounder who was a 150-pound sylph. Dr. Michaels' mortgage payments were assured. Yet, at the same time, the puppy-dog adulation of his patients and their extremely grateful and near-slavish behavior were incredible ego rewards. Everyone gained. Michaels got rich and got lots of ego strokes. The patients got thin. The insurance companies paid. The hospital had an assured clientele. And little guilt ensued.

After all, these patients were "sick." At least, they were hospital patients and that meant that they were "sick." It took surgery to cure their obesity. So this obesity had to be a form of "illness" and not the result of gluttony. Not so—but it made for a good rationalization. And the superobese patients were *not* predominantly female; the number was divided equally between men and women. Sometimes there were more male patients than female. While we have no accurate figures as to what percentage of the population—male or female—is three hundred or more pounds, it seems that men are more likely than women to seek a surgical cure for superobesity. It may be that the superobese female can loll or roll around her house, but a grossly obese man is incapable of earning a living and must somehow seek a quick and sure cure. In this case the cure is surgery.

Another explanation for the popularity of the jejunal bypass is purely psychological and somewhat Freudian. In their hatred for their bodies, the superobese seek ways to punish the ugly flesh that makes them miserable. Searching for a sympathetic listener and looking for a knife-happy surgeon to slice their bodies, they find someone who is willing to oblige their masochistic whims. Once more we can see the puritan ethic at work. If a superobese person suffers the pains and tribulations of severe surgery, endures postoperative trauma, lives through months and months of constant diarrhea, and adjusts his/her work schedule to bowel demands, then beauty will result. And it does.

Even though the superobese are nearly a caricature and truly an exaggeration of every overweight or overanxious beauty seeker in the United States, their saga is repeated by many—if not most—of us day after day. Diuretics. Diet pills. Diet doctors. Electrolysis. Dermabrasion. Freckle removers. Skin bleachers. Hair straighteners. Hair curlers. Tattoos.

Tattoos! Yes, that is the current fad. Although tattoo parlors reek of sleazy waterfronts and cheap bars, nice ladies and zingy college girls are joining the ranks of sailors and marines who proudly display their tattoos. The fad began with the popularization of Janis Joplin's heart-shaped tattoo just above her ankle. Now a teenie butterfly beneath the left breast or a discreet rose inside the thigh is sexy and smart. None of your gigantic snakes intertwined with banners proclaiming ''Mazie'' or ''Love to Mother'' for our current-*courant* ladies of style. No matter if it hurts. No matter if you may get an infection or hepatitis from a dirty needle. The point is to be a little ahead of everyone or at least, and for God's sake, within the mainstream of what is currently the in thing to do. Pain is incidental. Or, as we have seen previously, pain may be essential to enjoying the masochistic experience. Beauty is sort of hedonistic. However, if it takes pain to be beautiful, then everything is O.K.

It sure is painful to have electrolysis. Hair follicle by hair root, each individual unwanted ugly hair on upper lip, brow, cheek, or leg is burnt and yanked out. A current fad among gay men is to have the beard removed root by root and thus have a silky smooth baby's-bottom-like skin. And it costs thousands of dollars. Not to mention the loss of sleep and burning pain and excruciatingly long sessions at the "salon." Supposedly it is worth it. Just as supposedly it is worth it to have a woman's excess hair on arms and legs removed by wax treatments. Wax treatments are exorbitantly expensive in the United States, but both cheap and commonplace in Europe and Latin America. I first met arm and leg waxing in Mexico City and thereafter endured the pain every time I went anyplace in Latin America. Sometimes I was hard pressed to explain why I could not appear at a presentation or seminar, and never admitted to the fact that I was a wax junkie. But waxing is painful and may even be quite dangerous.

The client has to allow the hair to grow several weeks so that the treatment may be effective. While most Latin women and many southern European women have little or no compunction about bushy underarms or furry legs, it is embarrassing for a North American hairy brunette to wander about growing her excess arm/underarm/leg hair. It is very difficult for such a person not to grab depilatory or razor. So on to the salon, where ordinary paraffin wax is heated and then applied warm to the legs/arms/underarms/upper lip. Therein is the initial problem. Too cool, and the wax won't stick. Too hot, and you end up with second degree burns. Once the warm (hopefully) wax has cooled, it is stripped in long strands from legs and arm and lip. Yank. Pull. Scream! Yipes! As the wax is pulled off leg/arm/lip, the long strands of hair are yanked out by their very little roots. The advantage of this procedure is that it takes two to three weeks for the hair to grow back. Thus, as a furry brunette, I was spared daily shaving and cuts with a safety razor for those couple of weeks. However, in time, I had to add up the inconvenience of shaving versus the pain of wax treatments and brilliantly opted for inconvenience.

That's not to say that neither I nor millions of women like me have been able to forgo the constant battle of the eyebrow. Fashion dictates that eyebrows be perfectly and fashionably arched in the manner defined that year. Some years, the brows are thick. Other years, they are thin. You can even buy plastic shields with the "correct" brow shape cut out. You smack the plastic card up on your forehead over your own brow and tweeze happily away. Of course, eyebrows can be too light as well as too thick. For those who dye or tint their hair, eyebrow color is a dead giveaway even though hair roots may be covered. Salons will provide customers with eyebrow tints or bleaches. Even though this is a decidedly dangerous practice, women still risk blindness in order to have eyebrow and hair color match. Some chichi and not so chichi salons will also dye pubic hair. After all, if your eyebrows are light, your hair is blond, your arms and legs devoid of any dark hair, who is to know? Him! That's who! I am no expert on pubic hair dyeing, but have had some close friends who have endured this dubious experience. Their reports are varied, depending on their level of paranoia or callousness. I'm still inclined to think that like the eyebrow-tinting trip, anyone dyeing or bleaching hair on the genitalia is bound for one hell of a law suit.

Apparently women will endure anything from

whalebone corsets to stinging dyes in their never ending search for beauty. And beauty bought at a price—whether suffering, money, time, aching muscles, or all of the foregoing. For example, there is no medical or physiological evidence that massage tightens muscles or skin or loses inches or realigns bulges and bumps. Yet women at Elizabeth Arden's, presidents in the White House, and men at the local health club all lie peacefully under the soothing and poking fingers of the local masseuse/masseur. Only as an adjunct do I want to point out that I refer to real, honest-to-Betsy physical fitness massages and not the sexual gimmick front for prostitution massage parlors of recent ilk. Maybe the whole Rolfing technique derives from the pleasure-pain theory of beauty.

"Rolfing" involves a "Rolfer," amazingly enough. Rolfing is the procedure by which a Rolfer alternately beats, pummels, rolls, pinches, and generally torments a patient. The pain theoretically releases psychic energy. Since the Rolfer is also a trained psychologist/therapist, physical therapist, you are physically and emotionally cleansed at the same time. Sounds crazy but just as reasonable as anything else. Maybe we are indeed such an isolated and nontactile society that we have had to compartmentalize, institutionalize, merchandise, and package touching and physical contact. Esalen's hydrotherapy. T-groups. Encounter sessions. Primal scream. Holding and touching for $25 per session, please. They all add up to people needing to be touched for psychological and physical reasons. There again we have come full circle to the psychological-sexual-social aspects of fashion and style.

From painting one's face to cosmetic surgery, to simple massage, to Rolfing, we see that fashion, beauty, style, and sex are all terribly and terrifyingly intertwined.

What a weird and wild comment on modern America that we have to pay instructors for the privilege of being touched and felt. Always remembering, of course, that it is nonsexual touching. But touching just the same. We don't have a family priest or friendly minister, so we go to the local guru-shrink—your friendly family psychiatrist. It's as though we are indeed living in bubbles of plastic, afraid to feel or see. Treatises and tomes on the inner-directed person or the outward-directed person seek to analyze modern men and women. And we are probably the outer-directed people of such learned treatises. We get our values, instructions, mores, patterns of behavior, and modes of acting from *other* sources. We enjoy sports vicariously. We watch rather than participate.

We learn and watch with the mad little black box in our living rooms, dens, bedrooms, and kitchens. Big Brother is not watching us; we are watching Big Brother. Social scientists and media experts tell us about television's pernicious and vicious impact—but we're really not sure what level of intensity that impact has. Leaving aside the violence on television and its influence on children, let us look at how millions of people—and particularly and especially women—involve themselves and live lives of adventure courtesy of the tube.

6 Flickering Tube

Nearly eight million Americans know that the finest neurosurgeon in the United States is Dr. Nick Bellini, the greatest internist is Dr. Matt Powers, and they both work at Hope Memorial Hospital located on NBC. As a veteran of many years of viewing the tragedy-laden episodes of *The Doctors,* I have my doubts about the ability of Hope's staff to deliver good medical services because they are so busy with sundry illicit affairs, premarital pregnancies, and multitudinous divorces. My worries over the inefficiency of Hope Memorial's staff has reached such proportions that I wear a metal identification bracelet that, instead of a warning in big red letters reading "Diabetic" or "Sulfa-

Allergic,'' says, ''Don't Take Me to Hope Memorial Hospital!''

Farfetched? Hardly. Millions of viewers become intimately involved with the lives and problems of their favorite soap-opera heroes, heroines, and assorted villains and villainesses. About seven million people watch the leading shows each afternoon. Soap operas now have their own Emmy awards. Fan magazines print letters from viewers who worriedly inquire about the personal lives of stars, threaten mass defection should Mark marry Susy and leave Mamie, weep over the death of a special character, and pout when an actor is replaced.

Convoluted plots test the viewer who must keep at least three story lines disentangled at once. For the soap-opera buff it is relatively easy, particularly if she watches on Mondays and Fridays. On these days, loose ends from the previous or current week are unraveled or partially straightened out. Characters sit down over their ubiquitous cups of coffee or else have interminable telephone conversations, thereby filling the viewer in on the past few weeks of murder, mayhem, incest, and garden-variety perversion. As she immerses herself in the illusory world of soap operas, chimera substitutes for reality, her home becomes instant theater filled with salacious enchantment.

Soap operas are a uniquely American mode of entertainment. *As the World Turns, General Hospital,* and *Days of Our Lives* are direct descendants of radio's *Our Gal Sunday* and *The Romance of Helen Trent,* and the silent movie thriller *The Perils of Pauline.* Soap operas possess a plethora of useless dialogue worthy of the worst Dickensian serial. But the real antecedent of modern-day soap operas is the medieval morality play.

Strolling players wandered throughout Europe performing plays representing the seven cardinal sins. Like carvings beneath choir seats or hidden under cornices, morality and pornography melded together in the morality play. Ostensibly, actors portrayed the horrors of sin and the punishment of the damned, but actually audience passions warmed more when consciences were pricked by these graphic, lascivious peep shows. Eternal damnation seemed a petty price to pay for such alluring temptation. Alas, the pleasure was momentary and only vicarious, for townspeople, villains, serfs, and servants had little chance of gaining the minutest access to the most innocuous of transgressions. Their world was brutal, vicious, and dull, with every moment dedicated to staying alive, except for those rare instances of standing in the churchyard watching the wandering players.

So, too, does the modern soap opera appeal to the baser instincts of the average-woman-in-the-kitchen who, in all likelihood, does her afternoon ironing in front of her television set. At the same time, while titillating her daydreams, the chaos and affliction of afternoon TV makes the viewer's dull life seem well ordered and safe by comparison. For example, at one point on *General Hospital,* with seventeen major characters, there are four divorces, two premarital pregnancies, four illicit affairs, two male drug addicts, one male alcoholic, one male amnesiac, one male prisoner, and one female mental-hospital patient. Intellectuals sneer at soap operas, but 58 million viewers attest to their abiding popularity.

The Guiding Light has been on the air for nearly forty years. Actress Mary Stuart has played twice-widowed, twice-blind, and once-pregnant Joanna Tate on *Search for Tomorrow* for twenty-five years. With such a long run it is hardly surprising that Mary Stuart's professional and private lives impinge on each other. The first time that Mary Stuart was pregnant and Joanna Tate still unmarried, the cameramen shot her from behind furniture and from the neck up. When an eight-months pregnant Mary Stuart went shopping for a wedding dress to be used in the sequence of Joanna's first marriage, Mary reports that clerks sniffed their disapproval and called her "dearie," never "madam."

While Mary-Joanna received a little censure for being supposedly unwed and pregnant, Eileen Fulton, who plays Lisa Shea of *As the World Turns,* suffers more public discomfort than any other soap-opera star. Lisa Shea is the bitchiest of soap-opera bitches and is unalterably hated by seven million fans of the program. Eileen fled in terror from the appliance section of a large department store after watching a taped segment of her show and listening to women customers mutter how much they hated Lisa and wanted to kill her. On another occasion, a woman walked up to Eileen Fulton and asked if she were Lisa Shea. When Eileen replied yes and began searching in her purse for a pencil in order to give the woman her autograph, the fan began to beat Eileen with *her* purse, all the while screaming how dreadful Lisa Shea was. Eileen Fulton thinks she earns every bit of her $50,000 a year salary because of incidents like these and the time she nearly died on camera.

While Lisa Shea was supposedly fighting for her life in an oxygen tent, Eileen Fulton was too. The oxygen tent used on the show was completely zipped up in the back, but no oxygen was being pumped into the tent. As Lisa-Eileen coughed and strained for breath inside the big plastic bag, one of the stagehands crawled along the floor out of camera range and unzipped the back of the oxygen tent. Not only was there no thought of stopping the show, but Eileen and the director were pleased by mail from doctors and nurses about Lisa's condition. One doctor even wrote that Lisa was about to die because her fingernails were turning blue; he advised using penicillin and, should this fail, he suggested calling in another surgeon to do a tracheotomy.

Art, life, reality, fabrication, and the twilight zone become intermingled sometimes, and it is very hard for the average housewife to tell truth from fancy on television's phantasmagoric landscape. In the soaps (and to some extent, as we shall see, in nighttime TV) the ''worst'' aspects of a female value system are promulgated. Afternoon soaps foster an ideology based on female passivity, ineptness, and subservience. Married women bewail their barrenness and often have nervous breakdowns or, like Audrey on *General Hospital,* will actually steal a baby to make up for not breeding. Motherhood is the most important role for a woman, regardless of her education. Dr. Althea Davis, Dr. Maggie Powers (*The Doctors*), and Dr. Laura Horton (*Days of Our Lives*) have each attained the highest status-ranking on the North-Hatt scale and are full-time working professional women holding down positions of authority; yet these independent women manage to get themselves into the damndest messes from which only strong, brave, intelligent males can extricate them. The moral: Flibberty-gibbet females must be rescued by omnipotent males.

Two-dimensional soap-opera character development further reinforces cultural stereotypes of female passivity. A soap-opera heroine is acted *upon*. She is raped, divorced, abandoned, misunderstood, given drugs, and has endured mysterious diseases. More females than males in the soap opera go mad, have brain tumors, and die.

The female "sick role" with all its assorted bag and baggage of hypochondriacal symptoms is portrayed with antiseptic frequency on Sudsville. Soap-opera leading ladies never get simple influenza but suffer from obscure and wonderful diseases like *syringomelia, myasthenia gravis, subacutebacterialendocarditis, meningitis,* sundry brain tumors, not to mention that perennial favorite, *amnesia*, or its close runner-up, *partial amnesia.* From the medical thesaurus the writers deliberately select the most exotic illnesses, not only to awe the ladies but also so as not to alienate the majority of fans. However, recently soaps have departed from their love affair with subacutebacterialendocarditis and other multisyllabic illnesses and have gingerly approached the subjects of cervical and breast cancer. The overwhelming approval of fans and their personal involvement in Jennifer Brooks's (*The Young and the Restless*) mastectomy promises somewhat greater veracity in the future.

But important matters such as amnesia, partial amnesia, rape, murder, incest, and out-of-wedlock pregnancies are what really have center stage at all times.

Sin in the afternoon is played out against a lily-white, middle-class WASPy backdrop. Or at least the WASPy setting as the writers imagine it to be and the viewers want it to be. Silver tea services and book-lined libraries are sure symbols of upper-middle-class status. Sudsville heroines arise in the morning fully clothed with their eyelashes on straight and their Saks dresses unmussed. Husbands like Dr. Tom Horton (MacDonald Carey) of *Days of Our Lives* spend hours over the breakfast table talking to their wives. Of course, the moral is that if every wife looked like Mother Horton, her husband would stick around too. Mother Horton has never been seen slumping around in a chenille housecoat with fuzzy slippers and rollers in her hair. (For that matter, no soap heroine, good or bad, has ever been seen in the chenille-housecoat/fuzzy-slipper outfit that is an early morning uniform for most American housewives.) Not only do blondes have more fun but they have more sorrow on the afternoon soaps. Witness the number of blond heroines, like Drs. Althea Davis and Maggie Powers and Nurse Ryker. The women are blond and beautiful and the men are handsome and brave.

WASPy in format, Protestant in intent, and puritanical in morality, the afternoon soaps grind out their ethical message. All crimes will be punished. Retribution will strike down the most secretive and recalcitrant of sinners. Certain subjects such as homosexuality, lesbianism, and cannibalism are taboo, and although the soaps are sadomasochistic, the whip-and-chain crowd never appears on camera.

Whether any of soapland's characters *meant* to commit a crime (or sin) has no bearing on its final outcome. Whether the sin be of omission or commission, intentional or *deus ex machina*, disaster will follow. Nowhere is this rule followed more explicitly than in the case of sexual transgression.

All women and girls who engage in premarital or extramarital sex, through seduction, stupidity, or rape, will end up pregnant. Dr. Karen Werner, Nurse Ryker, Nurse Simpson of *The Doctors,* and poor unfortunate Dr. Laura Horton (who was raped by her brother-in-law, Dr. Bill Horton) are testimonials that pregnancy is the ultimate result of illicit intercourse. We pause and wonder why so many doctors and nurses are seemingly ignorant of basic contraceptive techniques and hope that these same.doctors and nurses *never* work in a Planned Parenthood clinic. Yet, to the pregnant blue-collar wife who is expecting her third unplanned baby, it is comforting to know that lady doctors and nurses get caught too.

Sudsville heroines who are legally or illegally pregnant give rise to a birthrate on afternoon TV that is eight times as high as the United States birthrate as a whole and higher than the birthrate of any underdeveloped nation in the world. This frenetic, rabbitlike parturition underscores the pronatalist attitude of TV writers.

Soaps don't worry about population explosion or problems of race prejudice or exclusionary clauses in country clubs: that's for the evening news. Sin is serious business in the afternoon. But that's because soapy life in the suburbs is so marvelously simple and clear-cut. Like the little girl with the curl, soap-opera characters are very, very good or very, very bad. A soap-opera *aficionada* must be as interested in snarled genealogy as any cultural anthropologist unraveling kinship structures of the Fuzzie-Wuzzies, since in-law and sibling relationships in characters relate to their personality types.

Goods are the ''tent-pole characters''—upon them is hung the story line. In *The Doctors,* good, kind, fatherly Dr. Matt Powers, administrator of Hope Memorial and world-famous internist, is the pivotal character who spends more time listening to his staff's tales of woe than he does operating or balancing Hope's budget. Mother Horton, of *Days of Our Lives,* is the strong motherly type to whom everyone pours out troubles over endless cups of coffee.

Bads are fun to spot and are usually women. The bitch-goddess is polar opposite to the long-suffering and constantly enduring Good. The scheming bitch is as much of a cultural stereotype as the madonna. Bads like Lisa Shea and Kathy Ryker typify woman as evil, woman in the thrall of Satan, and woman as seducer of men. While the viewer may be forced to wait months and even years, the bitch-goddess Bads finally do receive a kind of retribution. Rarely are they written out of the show, for their evil qualities make them such an interesting focal point of the story line and of audience hatred that it is hard to do without them. However, we must note that usually Lisa and Kathy's lies are uncovered and they too are unmasked by the men whom they previously duped. Obviously, the moral here is that not even thoroughly wicked women can trick men for very long.

The chameleon award goes to Rachel Davis Matthews Clark Frame Cory. Originally one of the bitchiest of the female Bads, Rachel has suffered through five marriages with only one slightly adulterous bastard. When *Another World* gave birth to *Somerset* (now defunct), Rachel's character began to change, and lately, since her December-May marriage to Mackenzie Cory, she has become a thorough martyr-misunderstood-madonna. But when Rachel was highly evil, she betrayed her mother, Ada. Every mother in the audience who feels betrayed by *her* daughter agonizes alongside Ada.

But just as important, Ms. Average can thrill to illicit love affairs and vicariously enjoy handsome men in the afternoon. Male sex appeal is critical to the popularity of soaps and soap stars. The Dorian Gray award of the year goes to Bill Hayes, whom most fortyish or fiftyish house-wives remember as Marguerite Piazza's singing partner on the 1950's *Show of Shows.* Hayes is the leading soap actor, earns $75,000 per year, made the cover of *Time* magazine, married his leading lady, and is forever gazing from the pages of fan magazines. Sex is good business for the soaps. The story is more important than logic.

Audiences become involved in their favorite story lines and grant a willing suspension of disbelief. Babies born on soaps a few years ago are now adults getting divorces—and their mothers still look like actresses in their thirties. One character was caught in a revolving door for seventeen days—depicted in flashbacks. One pregnancy lasted eighteen months. Housework simply doesn't exist.

Leading ladies *never* clean toilets, scrub floors, peel potatoes, or perform any of the mundane dirty tasks of housekeeping. Although it is hard to keep house in Saks originals and false eyelashes, the spic-and-span condition of the soap-opera homes combined with an absence of maids gives rise to the suspicion that products sold during intermission and station breaks account for such cleanliness. Following the pattern of portraying soap-opera heroines in a subservient role, TV commercials treat women as dummies. A NOW study indicated that nearly all TV ads show women inside the home working as housewives: 43 percent of women in ads were shown involved in household tasks; 38 percent were helping men; and 17 percent of the women were sex objects. Earth-shattering problems like clean toilet bowls, keeping leftover food palatable, and making dishes shiny are solved by an off-camera male voice or a man who flies through the window (meditate on that image for a while) or a man who visits the confused housewife. With a booming deep voice, like that of Zeus from Olympus, like that of Wagner's Siegfried passing through the Ring of Fire, an omnipotent male rescues a befuddled female from her dilemma and advises, ''Use Zappo to clean your toilet bowl, keep your food fresh, and your dishes gleaming.''

Mrs. Clean of Oshkosh, Wisconsin, may use Zappo, but Mother Horton never lifts a finger in her house. Mother Horton has never been seen cooking a meal, although gallons of coffee are consumed during the interminable catch-up conversations on *Days of Our Lives.* One of soap opera's great lines is, "You mean you're not going to eat breakfast!" One day someone is going to say, "Yes, goddamn it, I want breakfast. I haven't had breakfast for eighteen years and I think it is about time that you got off your can and cooked a meal for a change." Mother Horton would probably have a heart attack right on camera because her family has been eating at McDonald's and the Pizza King for the past eighteen years. She hasn't even unpacked her dishes and pots from the time she moved into the house as a bride.

Soap-opera heroines weasel out of housework and they and their menfolk take no part in community affairs. Occasionally, a minor rich-bitch character will sell tickets to a charity ball, but that's the extent of their community involvement. Note that no one is ever forced to buy tickets to attend a firemen's or policemen's ball. Actually, Sudsville is a truly dismal spot, where tragedy and desolation reign. In over fifteen years of watching soap operas, I have yet to hear a joke. Granted, only Lenny Bruce or Mort Sahl could make jokes about brain tumors or myasthenia gravis; still, a little pun might liven things up just a mite.

If things are tragic in Sudsville, they are disastrous from Kennebunk Port to Lubbock. Throughout the United States, women watch the soaps and become more and more miserable. Their misery is not just the result of overly profuse empathy concerning Maggie's brain tumor or Karen's partial amnesia, but comes from a profound sense of being cheated. Mrs. Average-Viewer knows that her home will never be as spotless as Mother Horton's, her face and figure never as perfect as Rachel's, her career never as exciting as Dr. Althea Davis' and her love life never as exciting as that of any of the harried premaritally pregnant heroines. Her husband isn't as lithe as Dr. Aldrich nor as attentive as Dr. Bellini. Her children aren't as well behaved as TV moppets and there are no dogs to wipe up after nor birdcages to clean in TV land. Sudsville is tragic because it serves as yet another vehicle to make the modern-day housewife unhappy with her own life.

The flickering half-light of the TV tube is a will-o'-the-wisp, beckoning and luring Middle American women to their doom. Every day the television set contrasts Louis XIV with Penney's best, Bendel's with Robert Hall's, Cartier's with K-Mart, and Bill Hayes with Harry the Plumber. It is not a pleasant comparison when the housewife looks around her home, peeks into the mirror, and glances at Harry. Everything is wrong. Nothing will ever be right. Better tune in tomorrow.

Or tune in tonight. Surely evening TV cannot be as denigrating as the afternoon soaps. Worse. At least in the afternoon morality plays, women do have numerous roles and contribute something sometimes to plot and character. Disaster is the mildest word that can describe evening TV.

A devastating in-house report in 1975 on Public Broadcasting[4] showed that in twenty-eight adult programs (panel, documentary, news, interview, and public affairs programs) there were two hundred males and only thirty-six females. And eleven of these twenty-eight programs had no women at all. Women were not ignored, they were overlooked. In *Theater in America,* 80 percent of the characters were male. While it appears at first glance that the wildly popular *Upstairs, Downstairs* drama favors women since 55 percent of the characters are women, 'tain't so. The majority of these characters are cast in traditionally feminine and subservient roles: maid, mother, etc.

If Public Broadcasting was not bad enough in 1974, its feeble attempts at recognizing International Women's Year in 1975 culminated in the shows *Jenny* and *Notorious Woman*. Jenny Churchill's sexual peccadilloes were overplayed in contrast to her political sagacity. Alistair Cooke, though, treated George Sand more kindly. While George Sand's tempestuous and bisexual love affairs took center stage, Cooke did give a measured account of Sand's literary contribution. On the other hand, Public Broadcasting did score a triumph of both dramatic and historical note with its analysis of British feminism late in 1975. But how strange that all these programs were British imports. Apparently American producers cannot stand to give women any roles in depth or portray historical heroines with any degree of veracity at all.

Male dominance. Male themes. Male voices. The Task Force Report on Public Broadcasting notes that *90* percent of the announcers promoting programs on Public Broadcasting are men. Just as in the afternoon the man from Glad, or the man from Tide, or the man from Peter Pan peanut butter, or the man from feminine hygiene spray gives instruction *to* the woman, so also on Public Broadcasting does a man instruct you on what to see. If Public Broadcasting—which at least gives lip service to liberalism and egalitarianism—has such a dismal track record, there is no reason to expect ABC, NBC, or CBS to portray women as other than silly, passive, dumb broads. And that's it with few exceptions.

The majority of shows portray women solely as help-mate, mother, secretary, general factotum, or seductress. Crusading lawyer Petrocelli has a faithful blond wife who types, drives a truck, and even has been known to lay bricks. Kojak, lollipop-sucking tough detective, doesn't have a woman cop or woman secretary in his precinct. Women appear in *Kojak* most often in the role of a tearful wife to whom Kojak has to break the news that her husband has been killed in the line of duty. Jim Rockford, of *The Rockford Files,* doesn't even have a secretary, although he does have one-night stands with old girl friends. *Barnaby Jones* has a former Miss America who portrays his daughter-in-law, secretary, aide, undercover agent, and confidante. That's what every man needs. *Marcus Welby* differs from the afternoon shows, because at least in the afternoon soaps there are some lady doctors. *Welby* only has nurses. And mostly one office nurse only. The list is endless and tiresome. Rare are the women who work. Only a few programs supposedly tout the new woman: educated, cosmopolitan, smart, witty, and perhaps happy.

There's the rub. Let's take a look at those shows with women protagonists and see what message comes through to males and females in the audience.

The Mary Tyler Moore Show is mother lode for spin-offs concerning women. Touted as a story of a sophisticated career woman, Mary Richards' misadventures in the mad city of Minneapolis are far from paeans to a well-adjusted young career-oriented woman. We get the impression that her job makes her more subservient to Mr. Grant, the TV producer, than the men in the studio. While Mary doesn't usually go to get the coffee, she rarely is shown writing, creating, or directing. Mary's primary occupation in life is dating, finding a date, looking for a date, dressing for a date, and talking over last night's date. Her relentless pursuit of a suitable man is all-encompassing and all-boring.

Mary's former neighbor, now married with a show of her own, is Rhoda. Valerie Harper's story is one of the Weight Watchers' successes. Originally a supporting comic character on *The Mary Tyler Moore Show,* Harper was decidedly overweight and so (off-camera) joined Weight Watchers. The wonders of thin. As Valerie Harper became thinner and thinner, her role as comic-foil and one-line artist became less and less believable. As she became thinner, she became less an object of fun. As a pretty girl a new future blossomed. So now Valerie Harper has her own show and her own torments. The weight gag is still carried out. Rhoda constantly remembers her fat days and wryly refers to her loneliness. Another reminder of Rhoda's fat past is her fat sister, Brenda. Brenda gobbles junk food incessantly, talks about dieting continually, and acts like the old Rhoda. Fat is funny on *Rhoda.*

Not so funny but infinitely tragic is the other spin-off from *Mary Tyler Moore, Phyllis.* Bitchy, fortyish, widowed Phyllis Lindstrom leaves mad, exciting Minneapolis to live with her deceased husband's mother and stepfather in San Francisco. Phyllis is seen trying to cope with dating; hunting for a job, although she has no skills;

keeping a job, although she is an upper-class doctor's wife snob and not used to taking orders; and desperately trying to combat excruciating empty hours. Maybe there is some wild explanation for *Phyllis'* ratings. Since Phyllis was so mean to her deceased husband, Lars, and nasty to both Mary and Rhoda, maybe she deserves her painful widowhood. Again the message is hardly subliminal but blatant: A man is necessary for survival—economic, social, and psychological survival. It's there every night.

Like the heroines of afternoon soaps, Mary, Phyllis, and Rhoda invariably get so entangled in sticky messes that some wise, powerful man has to bail each one out. Supercilious, overbearing Maude is no exception either.

Bea Arthur's portrayal of an upper-middle-class much-married pseudo-liberal is a delight to watch. Maude is the lady with the flowered hat who heads the PTA or Hadassah and who marched for causes when it was ever so popular to do so. Maude is tactless to the point of being mean. Her bumbling husband suffers under Maude's double-forked tongue. The neighbors grudgingly consent to listen to her diatribes. Why is she so popular? Because she is believable. She is not just a stereotype-come-to-life. She is every man's stereotype of what an emancipated woman would act like if only given half the chance.

Now Sgt. Pepper Anderson, portrayed by lithe Angie Dickinson, is quite another woman. Or is she? Elegantly pant-suited, carefully coiffed, security-ticketed, and husky-voiced Pepper is the one police detective who works with a Mod Squad group of cool dude po-leece. Pepper is smart and, although sensual, usually is portrayed as asexual or with no social life whatsoever. Invariably she will work in disguise as an undercover agent in the role of prostitute, dancer, or narcotics addict. Episode after episode she bravely works alone—even though wired for sound with microphones—and goes into traps with mad-dog killers. Zap! At the ultimate moment the mad-dog mob killer discovers dummy Pepper's ruse and is just about to kill her when the boys of the Mod Squad break the door down and save their pretty partner. Fade-out with Sgt. Pepper Anderson sobbing her relief in the arms of strong, tough, and supercapable Sgt. Bill Crowley. Women's lib loses again.

And the list continues with boring frequency. Women are portrayed as supporting actresses in traditional "feminine" roles. The ads portray the woman as housekeeper and sex object. Clairol is one of the few advertisers that show active, busy, educated, and reasonably nonneurotic women. The Tang ads are simply portrayals of Ph.D.'s in science who more than incidentally are mothers and serve their children Tang—because that's the astronaut's drink. I would hope that a Ph.D. in biochemistry could come up with a better reason than that.

Women who supposedly are articulate remain dummies on the flickering gray screen. Public Broadcasting's Report is right: Women are not denigrated; they are ignored. Where are the women hosts? Women predominate exclusively in the nicey-nicey artsy-craftsy programs of needlepoint, sewing, cooking, yoga, and exercise. Occasionally there is a semiliterate women's-libsy kind of program with depth or a reasonable imitation thereof aimed at women. But that's still sandbox television. Barbara Walters, Connie Chung, Cassie Mackin, and a few consumer affairs commentators are the reigning queens of television news. Most producers feel that a woman reading the news is not as effective or as believable as a man, and to date Walters on ABC has not changed that notion.

Thus it is that television is a dire desert for women. Voice-overs, hosts, stars, advertisements—all aspects of television ignore or play down woman's role as active participant in government, education, business, economics, and international affairs. Why not? The power plays of networks and producers are in the hands of men. Producers, directors, and to a great extent writers (excluding soap operas) plus technicians and engineers are predominantly and singularly male. Men write, direct, produce shows about men. Sensitivity to women cannot be expected by dominant macho males. It *is* a conspiracy. Males bound by cultural stereotypes wrought by centuries of myths and menopausal mothers continue showing women as silly ninnies. What's more, men and women apparently enjoy this depiction. For many women their reading matter reflects their mordant interest in soap operas, soap-opera stars, and media personalities from the wobbling tube. For those who refuse to admit being soap-opera or television junkies, the well-thumbed fan magazines in the chic salons attest that somebody (or many somebodies) is madly interested in television media gossip.

But the world of women's magazines is another matter. Magazines *for* women contain those topics that editors *think* women are interested in. A wild jungle untrod by male readers—but organized and manipulated by male editors—the women's magazine empire is a cutthroat maze.

7 Pulpy Passion

Puritanical in ethic and sexist in content, women's pulp magazines are sure-fire sellers. Grinding out their two- or three-syllable first-person stories of sordid sexual entanglements, swift retribution, penance, and a silver lining in the darkest of clouds, confession magazines endure and prosper. In an era when near institutions like *Look* and *Life* have disappeared from newsstands, the success of potboiler confession magazines cannot be ignored. *True Confessions, Modern Love,* and *Real Romance* are hardly big sellers compared to *McCall's* or *Woman's Day.* But *True Story*'s circulation is nearly double that of *Cosmopolitan*; and the combined circulations of Secret Romance Group, My Romance Group, and KMR Romance Group are higher than those of the slick, expensive fashion dictators, *Vogue* and *Harper's Bazaar.*

Women's pulp magazines continue because of their appeal to a forgotten but very large segment of North American women. Nearly one-quarter of confession-magazine readers have grade-school education or less, nearly two-thirds are married and under thirty-four years of age, while well over 80 percent are lower and working class. In all fairness, confession magazines probably reflect the actual sociological-demographical outline of the major-ity of United States women more accurately than do the reader profiles of the middle-class, high-school-educated, over thirty-five, married suburbanite *Woman's Day* reader or the young, college-educated, swinging-single, or pseudo-sophisticated young-married *Cosmopolitan* reader.

Based on over fifty years of publishing experience, the Macfadden-Bartell Women's Group (*True Confessions, True Story, True Romance, True Love, True Experience, Photoplay, Motion Picture, T.V. Radio Mirror,* and *Silver Screen*), with the assistance of sociologist Lee Rainwater's survey research, developed a statement of editorial policy that both analyzes its audience and stands as a credo for lower-class women's pulp magazines. Stating that its audi-ence is composed of wage earners or working-class women, the editorial policy proclaims that "the readers . . . reject the more sophisticated attitudes and approaches of middle class life." Rainwater's report further indicates that the typical reader of the Macfadden-Bartell magazines re-sponds emotionally rather than logically. Because she is so emotionally involved in the stories she then is able to find a solution to her own problems. Given such an editorial policy it is no wonder that the stories are so silly.

Pulp editors and writers seem to be convinced that lower-class women are passive ninnies. Heroines are borderline hysterics, neurotics who fight back tears, give in to tears, sob, gulp, choke, and break down. These women have good reason to cry, for they have managed to get themselves into horrible situations from which only strong handsome males can extricate them. A line-by-line analysis of thirty-seven stories from four different magazines showed that in 70 percent of tales, men resolved difficulties wrought by female idiocy. Male supremacy not only triumphs in confession magazines, it is a cultural imperative.

Well aware that women's liberation threatens male dominance and indeed the whole concept of male-female relationships, most short stories referring to women's liberation contain a reactionary message that the subservient but married lot is better than an independent but harried working woman's. In a *True Confessions* story entitled "Four Walls Do Not a Prison Make . . . ," Jo tells how happy she is *not* to be working and says:

> The only time I get the blues is when I read and hear some of the stuff put out by the women's libbers about how we gals should get out and work to broaden our horizons, keep up with our husbands, blah-blah-blah.

Jo recounts how the only thing that broadened for her when she worked as a secretary was her "bottom." Jo rushed to work in the morning and ran like a maniac all day long. She popped her pantyhose bending down to the file cabinets. She made her boss's coffee and ran his errands. She rushed back home to throw together a meal of "just hamburger" because she "wasn't up to preparing anything more creative." Jo resented her husband for not helping with the housework, but she felt that her husband had a right to sit in the living room with an extra cup of coffee while she was still "slaving in the kitchen." (Housework is woman's work and men should not share household tasks.)

Frustrated at trying to combine two roles, annoyed at her husband, frantic and harassed at her job, Jo finally quit when her boss asked her to type his son's school assignment. Jo delightedly burbles regarding her pregnancy, her book reading, oil painting, and finding the bottom of the laundry basket, even though she snidely comments, "Maybe I'm a cop-out to the libbers but I'm happy."

Jo can hardly be a "cop-out to the libbers" because she (and her creator) misunderstand the whole principle of women's liberation. Why didn't Jo tell her boss to make his own coffee? Why didn't she insist that her husband help with the housework? Why does her "happiness" have to be expressed in a pronatalist and parasitic existence? The message in this story comes across loud and clear— housework and babies are fun; a job is bad. Of course, given the struggle of working at boring, enervating jobs, most women would quit in a moment, if they could. However, most men would quit too, provided that they too had someone else to pay bills. According to confession magazine editors, the women's liberation message boils down to getting a job and neglecting the home.

This theme is repeated in another story entitled, "I've Had It with Women's Lib," and not too subtly subtitled, "A Homemaker Strikes Back." Even though Marcie delighted in her home and her home-baked cookies, her best friend, sophisticated and worldly Liza, made her feel guilty about being just a homemaker. Marcie got a job. She quickly learned it was better to be a homemaker than a tired typist pounding on the typewriter and suffering under a mean nasty boss. Worst of all, the children and husband tried to help Marcie with the household tasks. Dumb kids. Dumb husband. The beds were lumpy and the meals inedible. One day Marcie quit her job in disgust and returned home to find her children and husband parading in front of the house with placards reading "Children's Lib" and "Husbands' Lib." What a magnificent coincidence! Marcie realized then that her destiny lay in smooth beds and waiting on her husband and children.

Jo and Marcie project an editorial policy that comes across loudly. Don't cast aside your meal ticket for independence. No matter how unbearable your life may be, no matter what psychic pain you have to endure, a house in the suburbs is worth everything. In essence, pulp magazines underscore the women's liberation critique of North American marriage as nothing more than legalized prostitution.

Blue-collar women empathize with stories in which the heroine's major concern is to find a husband. Because blue-collar women earn poor salaries and because a female-headed home is headed for disaster, an employed husband is a necessary prerequisite for financial stability. Few pulp heroines are trained or skilled workers—like the majority of the readers. Blue-collar working-class women can easily identify with these heroines because the protagonists are employed in low-level, dull, uninteresting, and typically female occupations: waitress, secretary, saleslady. Of course, then, the message repeats itself—get a husband and keep him. But keeping him is always within the confines of married passion.

Sex is serious business in the pulp kingdom. Confession magazines are not "obscene" but contain a decidedly puritanical retributive morality. Whatever the transgression, punishment is direct and swift. All girls who engage in extramarital sex or premarital sex, or who accede willingly or unwillingly to rape, will end up pregnant or at least permanently branded as shameless hussies. Graphic descriptions of sexual intercourse are rare and usually employ such stock phrases as:

"He crushed me in his strong arms."

"Our bodies melted into each other and became one."

"I never knew that such delight existed."

In spite of their titillating subject matter, women's pulps describe sexual encounters in a most pedestrian manner: heaving breasts, cries of delight, shivers of ecstasy, and throbs of desire. Such stuff is hardly to be considered obscene except in a stylistic sense.

Because women's pulps supposedly concentrate on the sexual aspects of a woman's life, I analyzed fifty-three magazines representing eighteen different titles in order to determine the major themes recurring in women's magazines. Of the 651 features, I eliminated all doctors' columns, advice columns, recipe sections, letters to the editor, beauty tips, horoscopes, interviews with television or movie stars, and then analyzed the 489 remaining stories and novelettes.

Nearly a third of the stories are common garden-variety sexual topics, such as premarital sex, extramarital sex, or intercourse between two persons previously married to each other. There has, however, been a somewhat slight change compared to a few years ago. Recognizing changing sexual mores, confession magazines now allow young men and women to live together without ''benefit of clergy'' but with a tacit understanding that they will eventually marry each other in the last few paragraphs of the story; otherwise, the girl ends up pregnant, alone, ashamed, and abandoned.

Twelve percent of stories include medical-psychological-sexual problems, such as frigidity, impotence, vasectomies, feelings of sexual inadequacy after a mastectomy or hysterectomy, ectopic pregnancies, or a worried lady still a virgin after a year of marriage. With the help of a kindly and friendly old general practitioner, who probably makes house calls too, most of these problems are solved. Usually it is the woman who goes to her friendly G.P., and not the man. Thus, sexual problems are always the fault of the woman and rarely the man's.

The medium is hot and the message too. Short stories and full-length features consistently hammer home their reactionary messages. Women are emotional. Women must use their sexual wiles to succeed in life. Women must have a man to support them. Married sex is best. Any other sexual activity will harm the participant. Women cannot control their own lives. Women's liberation is evil.

It is interesting that confession magazine writers and editors seem to have made a Machiavellian pact with each other to twist and pervert the meaning of women's liberation. Since real-life factory women are demanding equal pay for equal work and day-care centers for their children, there is no reason to suppose that the basic principles of women's liberation are either foreign or inimical to working-class women.

What would happen if blue-collar women considered themselves as complete human beings rather than appendages and slaves of others? What would happen if blue-collar housewives and working women rejected the sexist philosophy of the pulps? If women didn't seek nirvana in clean toilet bowls, admen would disappear. If women ceased to believe in themselves as sex objects, the manufacturers of padded bras, crotchless panties, girdles with false rear-ends, and rhinestone pasties would go out of business.

But pulps are not the only women's magazines that put down the emancipated woman. Most of the middle-class women's magazines also exhibit a wild kind of ambivalence toward woman's emancipation versus woman's traditional roles. But all of them have had to change with the times. Most of the traditional middle-class magazines changed *after the fact*—rather than being leaders or harbingers of a new morality and new fashion.

Woman's Day, Family Circle, and *Good Housekeep-*

ing developed recipes for freezing dinners ten days ahead, twenty versions of hamburger casserole, and a host of easy-do-it recipes because a goodly majority of their readers work full- or part-time. *Redbook, McCall's,* and *Ladies' Home Journal* revamped their style and story content when it became quite obvious that their appeal to the muddle-headed multibabied housekeeper was all wrong. Ladies' magazines discovered that their audience had suddenly grown up—or become more aware—or never had been that muddle-headed anyway. Women were concerned over issues of abortion, equal pay, and sexual emancipation. And just plain ordinary garden-variety sex.

If you want sex in large doses, the ladies' magazines can supply it on demand: porno thinly disguised as doctors' advice columns, full-spread articles on abortion, hysterectomies, mastectomies, and transsexual surgery. You name it and the "nice" ladies' magazines cover it. While the pulp confession magazines have the *reputation* of being filled with porno yarns, the *Journal* and *McCall's* dress up their sex with respectable Ph.D.s and M.D.s. *McCall's*, the *Journal, Redbook*, and *Harper's Bazaar* all discuss at length the latest "new morality" or latest sex therapy in vogue. "Nice" ladies' magazines have discovered that sex sells and apparently offends few readers. *McCall's* even capitalizes on the generation gap in morality. Mother and daughter team Dorothy and Mary Rodgers answer questions on etiquette. Their answers to questions that Amy Vanderbilt would have spilled her tea over are a lesson in contrast between the generations.

One burning question is about sleeping arrangements.

A mother wrote to ask if her daughter, who shared an apartment with her live-in boyfriend, should sleep in the same bed with the boyfriend when they both came home for Christmas vacation. Mother Rodgers said no! Daughter Rodgers said yes! However, daughter Rodgers is nonetheless an upper-middle-class white matron and her stance on drugs, sexuality, morality, alcoholism, living-together, and divorce jibes reasonably well with Mama Rodgers'. That is not to say that this column is not at least a refreshing change from stock replies that were formerly handed out. As a matter of fact, the Rodgers column is more interesting in its subject matter than most of the lower-class pulp confession magazines.

Middle-class magazines and movie/gossip pulps do have two heroines in common—Jacqueline Bouvier Kennedy Onassis and Elizabeth Taylor Hilton Wilding Todd Fisher Burton Burton Warner. The sexploits, tragedies, illnesses, child and weight problems of these two women have probably been responsible for the decimation of thousands of acres of forest. You might imagine that the American female public would be sated with Elizabeth/Jackie. Apparently not. Inside exposés peeking into Liz/Jackie will pump up newsstand sales every time. The Jackie/Liz covers are hardly examples of good taste in either middle-class or blue-collar magazines. One pulp screams from its cover, ''The man that Lee and Jackie both loved at the same time,'' and the eager reader thumbs excitedly to the cover story. Surprise—Lee and Jackie both loved their father, Black Jack Bouvier! However, *McCall's* touts, ''The surprising New Life of Jacqueline Onassis.''

So what's so surprising? Jacqueline Onassis is working. That's surprising! Actually all the Kennedy women make good copy. Gallant Ethel and does she or doesn't she with Andy Williams? Poor, long-suffering Joan and does she or doesn't she like Jackie? Glamorous as they are, their private lives do remain essentially private. It's like trying to peek into a neighbor's window that is covered by a partially open venetian blind. You know something's going on in there but you can't really tell exactly what.

Everybody knows all about Elizabeth Taylor etc. Warner's private life, innards, penchant for chili, and passion for life. Pseudo-writer/psychoanalysts have psycho-analyzed Liz since she was twelve years old. *Everybody* knows about Elizabeth Taylor etc.'s father fixation, the many times she almost died on the operating table, her constant battle with the bulge, her grossly large diamonds, her yacht, and her wild arguments with Richard. Divorce, death, incredible wealth, and complete insouciance seem to be part of the Elizabeth and Jackie legend.

So the two reigning queens of women's magazines supply every dream-wish fulfillment for most American women. Wealth. Beauty. Jewels. Yachts. Couturier clothes. Travel. Ahah. The Protestant ethic wins again. We are all imbued with the knowledge that we can never be truly happy. You always have to *pay* for material goods with personal happiness. We all know that the poor are happy and the rich are miserable. Jackie and Liz just have to be miserable. They couldn't possibly unashamed-ly revel in their wealth. Jackie really still loves Jack. Liz really still loves Todd. And for those who subscribe to *hubris*, Liz's illnesses are just retribution for her sins.

But for sin-suffering-retribution and justly-being-struck-down-for-wickedness no one can beat the mass-media ghostly darlings: Judy Garland and Marilyn Monroe. Reams of analysis, reportage, recounting, first-person-I-knew-her-when stories have been cranked out over a period of too many years. The interesting method of the middle-class analytic/psychiatric authors is to describe "scientifically" and "dispassionately" the terrible things that drove Judy to her pills and Marilyn to her suicide. And it's really "those terrible things" rather than the ultimate demise of Judy/Marilyn that thrill the reader. Did Judy really participate in orgies on the MGM lot? Did Marilyn really have an affair with a high-ranking Washington politician?

But the aura of death and illness that hangs over Judy/Marilyn/Liz/Jackie is the Angel of Retribution. There is indeed a vengeful Jehovah who punishes these women for either their debauchery or their happiness. Therein lies the American puritan ethic. No one has any *right* to be rich, beautiful, popular, and beloved. Passion has to be countered by death. Life is not a soap opera; it is a bad Verdi opera. Safe in her midwestern nest or terrorized in her ghetto flat or bored on her farm or harassed in the typing pool, Ms. America receives comfort and consolation in knowing that Judy/Marilyn/Liz/Jackie all had to suffer enormously. Maybe then Ms. America's life is not really so bad or boring. After all, if the great glamour girls of the world are miserable, then that is the true existential meaning of life anyway. And we could continue on with examples of more pristine and proper ladies who also grace the pages of the middle-class magazines. Nancy Kissinger—who has ulcers and stomach problems. Betty Ford—and her saga of breast cancer. Lady Bird Johnson—and her loneliness.

But what do the middle-class mags offer as a balm to heal the hurt? If wealth, beauty, power, and popularity lead only and ultimately to tragedy, what is the magic route to happiness? Is there any? Again appealing to American folk wisdom, the ladies' magazines always have solutions. Casserole recipes. How to make curtains out of bed sheets. How to diet away your excess flab and become beautiful. If you work at your marriage, it will survive. If you work at decorating your home, your husband will want to stay in it. If you work at getting/keeping a svelte figure, you will get/keep/entice your husband. That's the underlying credo. If you steadfastly suffer, work, worry, and generally devote a great deal of energy to any task, virtue will be rewarded. That's why Judy/Jackie/Liz/Marilyn don't deserve happiness and thus are by definition not happy. They all were *born* rich and/or talented and/or beautiful. So they are doomed.

However, for Ms. America, who doesn't have the proverbial silver spoon or peaches-and-cream complexion, good old-fashioned technology and hard work will guarantee success. The definition of success is in terms of body shape, clothes, correct makeup, "in" hair styles, and current jewelry.

With their respective audiences in mind, each magazine touts its message. *Glamour* and *Mademoiselle* reach out for the recent college graduate and maybe—just maybe—the young married. *Vogue, Harper's Bazaar*, and to some extent *Country Life* deal with the stylish, modish, upper-middle-class soigné Neiman-Marcus, Bonwit Teller, a.ᴺᵈ Saks crowd. *Woman's Day* and *Family Circle* are for the pablum/typing-pool bunch, *McCall's* and *Ladies' Home Journal* for the solid middle-class civil servantry with solid incomes and stolid imagination. Yet as one thumbs through these magazines, the Seventh Avenue merchandisers with the "word" from Paris in combination with Madison Avenue touts and photographers obviously have covered the waterfront. A similar version of the same dress is featured in *Vogue* for $400; in *Glamour* for $195; as a Butterick Pattern in *Family Circle* for $50. Perfumes range from outrageous prices in *Harper's Bazaar* to soft little woodsy scents advertised in *McCall's. Country Life* advises its readers to go to the Golden Door; The *Journal* recommends your local health club; *Mademoiselle* suggests the local Y; and *Woman's Day* provides exercises to be done at home. The lyrics are slightly different, but everywoman is marching to the drum of New York fashion merchandisers. Yet it is interesting to note the variation in body size and type from magazine to magazine.

In accord with the dictum that thin means beautiful and thin means rich, *Vogue* and *Harper's* models are scrawny, no-chested androgynous creatures who look as though they just came out of Buchenwald. *Glamour* and *Mademoiselle* models are fresh-faced Anglo-Saxons with a little more meat on their bones—but they are still flat-hipped and have only a suggested bustline. The *Ladies' Home Journal* and

McCall's models, although still trim, are more buxom and contoured than models in other magazines. Similarly, models from *Woman's Day* and *Family Circle* pages are supposedly prototypes of chic North American housewives. And for truly buxom lassies, take a peek at the photographic illustrations for *Confession* and *True Detective* pulps. There seems to be an edict stating that the lower the social class ranking of the magazine the bigger the chest and hip measurements of the models. Obviously, the lower-ranked magazines don't have *fat* women—just bosomy, cheeky ones.

Even though there is this difference, the fashion advertisements and full-page feature spreads show that a certain type of body is necessary for draping the latest creation from Jonathan Logan or Halston. Properly accessorized and tastefully made up, the stylish young woman is ready. Ready for what? Why has she dieted and bumped her lumps away? Why is she spending money on gold chains, little hats, wide belts, thin belts, scarves, and chunky shoes? To be fashionable? Not really. The whole getup and the whole fashion game are predicated on the fact that being in style implies that the woman is prepared to accept her role as sex object. That's why female human plumage is more gaudy (at times) than male attire. The female is attracting the man. Success is defined by getting and keeping a man. The best way to get and keep said man is by first being a sex object in dress and damned sexy in the sack. And magazines help in the search for the big O.

Orgasm for orgasm no magazine can beat *Cosmopolitan.* Supposedly a magazine for swinging liberated females who work and engage in superb gymnastic routines in bed, *Cosmo* reads more like a *Field & Stream* manual on "How to Trap Your Man." Seductive cooking, seductive clothing, seductive apartment decorating, seductive toilet-bowl cleaning—all sock a message across that a woman *must* have a man. A man is a meal ticket. A man soothes loneliness. Sex is the means to get the man. Of course, if incidentally the woman enjoys herself, so much the better. Enticement and entrapment are the orders for the day. No wile, no trick, no artifice, no trap is considered unworthy if the prize attained is a male with a good Dun and Bradstreet rating. How to trap Mr. D & B is what makes *Cosmo* one of the hottest properties in the publishing business.

Today's *Cosmo* is a far cry from the dull, rather semi-intellectual *Cosmopolitan* of short stories and an occasional recipe interspersed with child-care columns that I remember my mother reading. As my morality has departed from my mother's, so also has *Cosmo* grown up too. Helen Gurley Brown took over a sick, ailing magazine and infused it with the "Sex and the Single Girl" ethos. She knew from firsthand experience that sex is not only fun but writing about it can be financially rewarding—especially for publishers. The courtesan ethic hit the newsstands with a gangbang. The liberated woman didn't sleep around town; she had interesting relationships. The working girl didn't have an affair with her boss; she just was overcome by the passion of the moment. If there were no eligible males in the readers' lives, *Cosmo* told readers where and how to find them. By the way, the answer is to move to Alaska or Houston and wear sexy clothes.

Interestingly enough, sexy, clinging, plunging clothes are the hallmark of *Cosmo* covers. Every (repeat *every*) cover of *Cosmo* has had a beautiful model with diving décolletage. Therein is a capsule tale. If *Cosmo* is the magazine for the swinging young married or nonchalant recent divorcée, and if *Cosmo* supposedly leads the magazine industry in its free-wheeling approach to woman's sexuality, then why a repeated cover of a woman with her boobies hanging out? If you look at a series of *Cosmo* covers from several months, you are immediately struck by the incredible *sameness* of models, faces, poses, and chests. Variations occur with color of model (an occasional very Caucasian-looking black) and color of dress (red for Valentine's Day and green for Saint Patrick's). And each model's vapid stare reflects an unimaginative content. As the covers are similar month after month, so too is the content. Horoscopes concentrate on love possibilities and marriage dates. Recipes are quickie gourmet items with aphrodisiacal properties. Clothes are (of course) clinging and breast-exposing. Diets show how to obtain the curvy body that supports the clinging clothes. Doctors' columns and reports excerpted from the latest sex manual advise readers what to do and how to do it when the curvy body with the clinging clothes has enticed the poor unsuspecting son-of-a-bitch into the (tastefully decorated) bedroom. In short, *Cosmo* is little different from *McCall's*, the *Journal*, or even *Redbook*. How to help a man attain an erection is scientifically, and tastefully, discussed also in *McCall's* and the *Journal*. *Redbook* regularly and scientifically surveys its readers on sexual mores of the times.

Unlike the *McCall's* genre, *Cosmo* rarely has articles on child care, although an article on divorced mothers and their sex lives did deal with the burning questions of baby-sitters and sleep-in lovers. However *Cosmo* is not an exception to the women's magazine business. *Vogue* and *Harper's Bazaar* both pretend that children do not exist. Sometimes the fashion mags feature exclusive and very expensive maternity clothes. And periodically slender society matrons pose with the latest from Saks' mother and daughter outfits. However the general consensus at *Vogue* and *Harper's* seems to be (1) that children are never seen, or (2) that they are always well behaved, or (3) that they ought to be popped off to boarding school.

Since *Cosmo* readers probably don't have enough money to send their kids to boarding school, *Cosmo* devotes many pages on how *not* to have children. Birth-control discoveries are the hottest fad in *Cosmopolitan* as well as *McCall's, Ladies' Home Journal*, and *Good Housekeeping. Cosmo* is not the only women's magazine that has discovered that tasteful, scientific physiological articles are supersexy. Because no matter how you slice it, a tasteful scientific discussion of genital organs, masturbation, lubrication, and interesting gyrations during intercourse is still just a wee bit lascivious.

But the one item that *Cosmo* has that no other staid magazine has is Florence King. Rollicking, Rabelaisian King is one of the wildest writers around, with one of the sharpest wits. She gives credence to the fact that some women (and at least one woman writer) see the funny side of sex. Florence King may not be the muse but certainly is

the court jester of the sexual revolution. King narrates all
her tales in first person and they usually involve painful
humiliation in light of sexual liberation. Growing up WASP
and southern, deflowered in the 1950's, living alone, enduring a series of nonentity lovers and worrying over pregnancy and multiple orgasms, King speaks for women in
their late thirties who are betwixt and between generations.
Too old for the swinging seventies and too young to settle
for complacency, this age group can't decide whether to be
shocked at the devil-may-care attitude of today's youth or to
lose all propriety and join them with abandon. King has
joined the swingers and her bitter-funny personal vignettes
provide both pity and a gasp of recognition. But Helen
Gurley Brown was not the first to recognize King's zany
humor. King came to prominence via *Playgirl* and *Viva*.
King's kookie, outrageous humor was well suited to the
Viva audience and apparently transferable to the *Cosmo*
crowd.

Actually the success of *Playgirl* and *Viva* blew most
magazine editors' sense of propriety and even sexologists'
concepts of female erotica. With Kinsey, one cardinal rule
had developed about female sexuality—women did not
enjoy erotica. Of course few people took into account that
most if not all erotica was male erotica. Besides, women
were well conditioned that nice ladies didn't enjoy erotica—only bad ladies did. But those were the days when nice
ladies didn't enjoy sex either—real sex or vicarious sex. As
more and more women became orgasmic, aware of themselves and aware of their own bodies, their prurient interests
were pruriented. *Viva* and *Playgirl* filled the bill.

Magazines contained full nude male centerfolds with male genitalia exposed for all the world to see, and sales mounted.

Another tenet fell before the onslaught of cold fact. Women enjoyed looking at pictures of nude men. Women enjoyed ribald and off-beat-off-color jokes and cartoons. Of course that is not to deny the distinct and obvious possibility that *Viva-Playgirl-Foxy Lady* audiences are not solely female. Indeed some if not many of their readers are male homosexuals who also drool over the male centerfolds. Unfortunately many of the male centerfolds are dreadful disappointments. Models' penises shrink on-camera and their pubic hair is decidedly scanty. Rather than being exciting types to stir the hormones of Ms. America, the male models look more like shorty gigolos who really do need the money from posing. But these male nudes are a far cry from *Cosmo*'s Burt Reynolds centerfold with Burt's elbow modestly hiding what all Ms. America was simply dying to see. And never got to see. Only Dinah Shore really knows. Sexploitation apparently then works both ways.

Ms. magazine was originally designed as a political statement and answer to rampant sexism. Gloria Steinem and company defiantly refused to accept ads for vaginal deodorants, but accepted perfume and hair spray ads. Now *Ms.* tries valiantly to be all things to all women in the women's movement and just as valiantly fails. Not gay enough for gay women. Not straight enough for straight women. Attacked for being too conservative and also too liberal, *Ms.* somehow limps along. It too is a magazine success story because of the outpouring of support in subscriptions whenever Steinem and her crew make an appeal for additional readers or paid-up dues.

At one time it was a mark of sophistication for liberated women to discuss the current issue of *Ms.* But lately most comments seem to center around how *Ms.* is boring and often shrill. Writers of note and talent are interspersed with badly phrased articles. No wonder. *Ms.* suffers from mounds and mounds of unsolicited manuscripts. Notes appear in editors' columns explaining that *Ms.* tries to live up to its credo of helping all women in the woman's movement—and even sometimes outside of it—by reviewing all these manuscripts. It's an impossible task, and the editorial unevenness of *Ms.* underscores that fact. However *Ms.* does illustrate the underlying sexism of newspaper advertising, matchbook covers, employment pamphlets, and inequities of the law in its "Gazette" and "No Comment" sections. *Ms.* scrutinizes legislation for and against women, gives publicity to women writers, television workers, film makers, and even forgotten women—forgotten, that is, in the history books. Yet the faults of *Ms.* are in themselves reflections of divisions within the woman's movement. Where does sisterhood leave off and competency and talent begin?

In other words, if you are a woman, you're O.K. by *Ms.* standards. That is, you're O.K. if you are a creative type who is flying in the face of a male-dominated establishment, whatever that establishment may be—plumbers' union or medical school. That's the crucial point. You have to have your head on right and your politics O.K. according to the *Ms.* credo. *Ms.* does not speak to the married homemaker/housewife except to berate her. Woe betide the

woman who says that she likes her kitchen and her needlepoint and her children and her potted plants. If she
doesn't work at a creative, mind-fulfilling job, have a
homosexual liaison once in a while, engage in creative
adultery, and flout fashion—then she's still entrapped in the
sexual-bourgeois cult of Madison Avenue advertising executives. To a certain degree that analysis is correct. However, the credo of the woman's movement seemed to concern itself with "liberation." That is, men were to share in
housework and child care, and women were not to accept
alimony when their marriages broke up; and maybe marriage was a boring middle-class trap anyway. Be that as it
may, *Ms.* still gives off some strange messages that may
not say, "BUY! BUY!" but the message at least says,
"BELIEVE! BELIEVE!" The political or pop sociological
message gets all glommed up with 1960's lefty-trendy
rhetoric. *Ms.* survives and hopefully, with more experience
and with less in-fighting amongst the staff, has the possibility of getting better.

Ms.'s financial success—shaky though it may have
been at the best of times—showed *Redbook-Journal-
McCall's* editorial staff that times were changing and they
had better get with the times—or else lose a young, well-
heeled, and reasonably well-employed audience. Susy
Homemaker was going to work. Cathy College was not
getting married right out of college and settling down in
mortgaged suburbia. *Glamour* now even discusses birth
control, living together, and abortion without a blush. *Redbook* makes sex surveys. So the *Ms.* readers—or at least
those who were not fully committed and dedicated femi-

nists à la Steinem—have returned to their mother's favorite magazines. Women obviously still read women's magazines.

So now the message is still "BUY!" but in accord with the hectic life of wife/mother/housewife/employee. Short-cut recipes. Microwave ovens. Blow-comb hair styles. They all reflect a harried, hag-ridden, commuter-exhausted woman who now must be all things to all audiences. She must be successful in her job, a true child-care expert, glamorous and well-groomed, an impeccable housekeeper and gourmet cook. So she will accomplish all these things courtesy of the women's mags. Too bad that a banner of emancipation seems to cover up further slavery. It may be heresy, but the wonderful emancipated life doesn't seem to be so wonderful.

With sexy lessons from *Cosmo*, etiquette tips from *Glamour*, and the fashion savvy of *Mademoiselle* combined with *Vogue* comes the ultimate feminine success—a wedding proposal. The ultimate in a young woman's dream comes the day she buys her *Modern Bride* or *Bride's Magazine*. She peruses *Modern Bride* for china patterns, silver patterns, matching and contrasting linens, kitchen appliances, and the *pièce de résistance*—a wedding gown. A gown it is and a dress it is not. Page after page of gowns—long, short, expensive, inexpensive, brocade to homespun. Dresses for bridesmaids. Dresses for mothers of the bride and mothers of the groom. Blue lace-edged garters. Pillows for the ring bearer to bear the ring. Veils. Mantillas. A profusion and proliferation of cultural traditions, folkways of bygone tribes, Greek and Roman symbolism, and Madison Avenue hype with Seventh Avenue kitsch.

And of course the most truly pathetic advertisements are those touting Poconos honeymoon hotels. Ads proclaim the joys of breakfast in bed, heart-shaped indoor pools, heart-shaped king-size beds, champagne, and I suppose lots of lovely love. The ritualized honeymoon and its mass-produced passion meet in the Poconos. If you don't want to spend all your time "alone" as the ads euphemistically giggle, you can, in season, play tennis, enjoy the outdoor pool, ski, fish, shoot, ride horseback, steam in the sauna, play at archery, and eat gourmet meals. There must be some reason behind the sports *mens sana* ethic of these honeymoon resorts. Maybe if you are exhausted from playing tennis or swimming, then sexual inadequacies are unimportant. Or the sports complex provides an opportunity for the *macho* to further impress his new mate. Whatever the reason, the whole honeymoon-resort complex complete with heart-shaped beds gives pause for thought. And it is on the pages of the brides' magazines that the whole fruition of the feminine dream arrives.

But there is a worm amid the flowers of Elysium. While the majority of photographs in brides' magazines portray obviously young and (sort of obviously) virginal WASPy models, here and there you find a somewhat older and decidedly worldly looking model. She is (fortunately or unfortunately) the bride second-time-around. Maybe she isn't a bride because the word itself implies virginity and intimates a first marriage. But indeed we find that bride magazines slowly are beginning to admit that divorce and remarriage are facts of life. As such, those facts have to be taken into consideration by the market research analysts. More surprising are advice columns to women on alimony and child-support problems that the second marriage can expect to face. Compared to the pristine and obviously virginal and somewhat prissy approach taken by *Modern Bride* in the early 1960's, when I was seeking my perfect wedding gown, the advice columns are hotter than firecrackers.

Modern Bride and *Bride's Magazine* realize that they are dealing with a sexually aware, even though inhibited, generation. This group of men and women have been having prolonged intercourse over many years. Virginal white may be the approved color for wedding gowns but nary a virgin is walking down the aisles these days. M.D.s and research psychologists frankly discuss masturbation, lubrication problems, various positions during intercourse, "sexy talk," venereal disease, and current thinking on birth control. As a matter of fact, *Modern Bride* and *Bride's* seem to have a more straightforward and somewhat slightly more clinical attitude than the voyeurism of *Cosmo*. I remember *Modern Bride* in the 1960's advocating only a "lean back and enjoy it" ethic and never mentioning anal and oral intercourse. Times have indeed changed.

But after the honeymoon, back to the job. After gliding down the aisle and being photographed like a movie star, the bride deals with dirty dishes and dirty socks. After the wedding comes the rude awakening. "The honeymoon is over'' is a pitiful cliché to describe a relationship. And it is over the night that your best friend drags out her wedding book and softly starts to cry over how fat she has become or how miserable she is. For many women their wedding day is their only starring day. All eyes are upon the bride. All attention is focused on the bride. The wedding is a zenith. Life ever afterward is a nadir.

Therein lies the difficulty of mass media. Forever portraying a fantasy world where no pain, no sorrow, no death, no boredom ever intrude. Consumer consumption will assuage any and all problems if they do trickle in. If nothing else works, new clothes, new recipes, new sexual techniques, and new surgical ones, too, will soothe and correct. That's not to say that women's magazines are not making a somewhat pitiful attempt to remedy their past sins.

Given newspaper coverage of the dangers of the pill, the current controversy over abortion, and the public's ghoulish preoccupation with Mrs. Ford's mastectomy, magazines have sensed a trend. Some medical writers, like Barbara Seaman of *Woman's Day*, have taken singularly courageous stands against the pill and unnecessary female surgery. As public indignation increases against doctors, insurance fraud, and malpractice, magazine editors seem to be willing to attack or at least criticize formerly sacrosanct medical doctors. Yet we must note that magazines' editorial policy *follows* current trends and doesn't set them. Hem lines can go up or down at the airy wave of an editor's pencil. Hair styles are straight or wavy in accord with the desire of designers and photographers. But serious discussion of male or female medicine is rare indeed. No one expects *Mademoiselle* or *Glamour* to be as polemic as *Ms.*, but some sense of social conscience seems to be stirring between the glossy covers of women's magazines.

Admittedly the initial stages of the 1960's women's liberation movement were bloody scary to women's magazine editors. Betty Friedan spoke to women in their "comfortable concentration camps"—i.e., ticky-tacky suburban boxes—and dangled reality before their eyes. Drowning in advertising and seduced by promises, the woman herself was a zombie. Friedan's book told women not to buy the products and to cut through ties binding women fruitlessly to idiotic work. That was revolutionary. No wonder that the early 1960's saw women's magazines ridiculing leaders of women's liberation as "scruffy" and "mangy." The supposed bra-burning at Atlantic City's Miss America contest never took place. No matter. As far as mass media are concerned, it did.

Yet the women's movement did speak to and for a large proportion of American women. Silently and without too much clamor, women began to move back into the world of work and school. In spite of sociologists who predicted the downfall of Western European family life, and in spite of Freudian psychologists who muttered about castrating females, women began to pick up pieces of their lives and reorganize themselves so as to become full human beings rather than appendages. However, most women did not abandon fashion; they continued to visit the hairdresser, they continued experimenting with new kinds of makeup, and in general they did not abnegate all the feminine tricks, wiles, and fun aspects of fashion. When magazine editors took another look at the emancipated woman, dollar signs danced before their eyes.

Now editorial policy decrees that the working woman/mother/wife/divorcée or swinging lady about town is a good bet. She may not wear a bra, but does slink around in mat jersey or Qiana. Articles and features focus on brainy (and beautiful) successful women who are real-life role models. Editors carefully avoid Dr. Suzanne Schlump, Ph.D.—she of the oxford brogues, thirty extra pounds, and rumpled lab coat—and substitute Dr. Mary Smarty, M.D., who does brain surgery on her kitchen table while dashed in Arpège perfume and adorned with shimmering eye shadow. Sometimes I wonder if the new role models are not reminiscent of the Virgin Mary. To be wife, mother, and virgin is impossible, but the Madonna did it.

To be wife, mother, brain surgeon, gracious hostess, connoisseur of the arts, clothes horse, and champion skeet shooter takes a little time, but it can be done. Naturally some details are usually missing. Lady brain surgeons, sociologists, movers and shakers of industry (female variety) more often than not have full-time servants, live-in mothers, flexible schedules, superunderstanding husbands, and maybe kids in boarding school. That's a hard combination for a kindergarten teacher in Peoria to repeat. My nemesis is Dr. Tenley Albright, Olympic gold medal figure-skating champion, Boston surgeon, mother of three, beautiful, chic, thin, and happily married. Dr. Tenley Albright haunts my dreams. I can't figure skate and only dissected a frog in high school.

What is it that makes so many of us so very dissatisfied

with what others would consider good lives? The housewife wants to work. The typist wants to lose ten pounds. The lady psychologist wants to prepare gourmet meals. The woman social worker wants a new nose. Why? The answer can't be patently mass media pounding away—although that's a part answer. Is it the whole American ethos of forever living in the future? Next year I'll be finished with high school, and then. . . . Ten years from now the mortgage will be paid and then. . . . And then you end up with no dreams ever fulfilled and the sad realization that those were too many years wasted wishing, wanting, hoping, and fantasizing. Not dreaming but fantasizing. A fantasy can never be realized—but a dream may be somewhat conceptualized. Mass media spin dreams and speak to fantasy.

For men success is money, status, and power. What is success to a black man? According to Eldridge Cleaver, it is a white woman. What is success to a short, balding, unprepossessing little man? According to Hollywood, it is a tall, blond, overpainted chorine draped in mink. What is success for women? According to mass media, it is a wedding ring, a house, a silver pattern with coordinated china, and, if at all possible, a mink coat too. The rules of the male/female success game are that fat, bald, dumpy men can attain success, but fat, thin-haired, dumpy little women can't. If you are a woman, regardless of your profession—brain surgeon, housewife, typist, or sociologist—and you are plain or overweight, you are worthless. Beauty (or a reasonable facsimile thereof) in combination with good cooking, an impeccably clean home in suburbia, quiet children, plus the most important ingredient, a good, faithful, rich, sexually adept husband, all add up to female success. No matter what pages of what magazines, blue collar or white, there it is in black and blue and white and four-color full-page advertisements. Get yourself in shape and get yourself a man by any means possible.

8 Some Faint Glimmers of Sense

It's a wonder that any one of us survives with a modicum of sanity. Although she is already dissatisfied with her clothes and her body, the very fabric of Ms. America's life is made to seem dull by the media, assaulted by daily contrasts with the captivating activities of soap-opera heroines or protagonists of pulp magazines. Compared to the virile Greek gods of afternoon Sudsville, her own husband is a dull clod. Contrasted to the well-mannered, soft-spoken children in the daily dramas, her own are boisterous, uncouth animals. Her occasional and unimaginative bedroom gymnastics are scarcely as interesting as the sordid sex life described in the confession magazines. Just as we believe that we will never age, so we think that only small-nosed, nubile young persons with straight teeth can have any fun. Only young beautiful slim-hipped bodies can know the Joy of Sex. Skin flicks, educational sex films, and X-rated movies never portray chunky forty-year-olds engaging in rambunctious sexual activity, although there is one film about a lithe, sexy sixty-year-old. But thin means sexy, and fat means repulsive.

Weight Watchers Magazine publishes letters in its regular feature, "Letters to Jean Nidetch," which reiterate the fact that men find fat women disgusting. How can any man make passionate love to a lumpy, creepy glob of blubber? On the other hand, several authors contend that fat women are sexier than thin women. Fat women supposedly spend more time pleasing others than do selfish, dieting thin women. Not bothered by the pangs of dieting, the fat woman can devote her gluttonish self to bedroom romps. Fat women are orally inclined and like to engage in oral sex. Fat women are uninhibited partners and much more sexy than the constantly dieting thin woman.

Yet Abraham Friedman, M.D., contends that fat people are overweight because of a lack of sexual activity. Dr. Friedman does not prescribe reducing diets but rather counsels his patients to "reach for your mate instead of your plate." He points out that the average bout of sexual intercourse consumes approximately two hundred calories, increases breathing, decreases desire for food, and simply substitutes one basic need for another.

Movies, television, magazine and book illustrations tell us that only good-looking people have tempestuous love affairs. Alas, few of us are Ingrid Bergman or Gregory

Peck. Luckily all of us don't buy the mass-media message. Ugly people can have feelings of passion.

It is an interesting psychiatric-surgical problem determining how and in what manner a person's own conception of her/his body image affects her/his actions. The literature on obesity and cosmetic surgery is quite unclear as to this point. Some people use their body disfigurement as a defense mechanism and when, through surgery or diet, they become "normal," their behavior often becomes quite aberrant. For example, the person who is convinced that nobody likes him because he has a large bulbous nose decides to get a new nose. After surgery he finds out that people don't like him even though he has a small nose. He is simply and succinctly a nasty person. And sometimes when people no longer have a physical defect to blame for their lack of success or friends, their reactions may range from alcoholism to suicide.

That's not to say that people who have had facial scars disappear through skin grafts or women who have slimmed down courtesy of Dr. Atkins' diet do not experience a more satisfactory life. As a matter of fact, I have seen personality improvement go hand in hand with physical improvement. Some people are hostile and defensive because of a physical deformity. What's more, their hostility and mechanisms are justified. The boy with an ugly birthmark all over his face can't get dates. The overweight teen-ager sits at home while her girl friends go to the junior prom. When the birthmark disappears or the overweight no longer exists, dates and friends are much easier to obtain.

It is unfortunate but we do react to dress and body size.

One good reason why stereotypes persist is that there is usually more than a tiny bit of truth to justify their existence. Whenever I go to a conference of sociologists or psychologists, I never have to look for "my people." I look for the men in open-necked shirts with long beards and curling hair—those are the sociologists. The men with beards, Prince Valiant haircuts, and expensive suits are psychologists. Anthropologists are a breed apart. The men have scraggly beards and the women have long hair. Both men and women anthropologists wear ethnicky clothes from their latest field trip to Bolivia or Boola-Boola and lug green bookbags around from meeting to meeting.

Clothes and physical appearance are political statements. Dashikis and shark's tooth necklaces were *de rigueur* dress for young black militants in the 1960's. In the 1970's prescribed dress for the young black man is the Brooks Brothers' suit and only a genteel Afro. The message here is the young black has arrived, has decided to blend in with mainstream American society, has become part of the social fabric of upward mobility, and everyone knows it by his dress. Afros for blacks—beards for academics. The beard of male sociologists is contrasted with short clipped hair for army officers. While the army officer *must* keep his hair short by regulation, the male sociologist is almost as equally hamstrung. While few male sociologists will lose their jobs for *not* having a beard, the beard syndrome is still a strong precept among academics.

I have had strange experiences with male social scientists who are job hunting. These men come to my office for an interview looking as though dressed for a local rock concert. Often the candidates are really quite good, but their dress and standards of cleanliness leave a great deal to be desired. One time I told a young man to return the next day and I would take him to various offices for interviews. I tried to explain as subtly as possible that it might be a good idea if he wore a shirt, tie, suit, and shoes, rather than his sweater, jeans, and sandals outfit. He duly returned the next day dressed in a reasonable facsimile of my request. The only problem was he wasn't wearing any socks. I hadn't told him to wear socks! (By the way, he didn't impress anyone in the interview.)

So we continually rate people by their dress. Most middle-class women can give you an estimate within a few dollars of the cost of every dress worn by every woman who comes her way. Maybe that's why Rosalynn Carter's wash-and-wear syndrome was so refreshing. Or at least politically savvy. Rosalynn was not stylish. She was every woman in polyester. Rather than remake her image in the Kennedy tradition, she traipsed about the country in her wash-and-wear best. She became the darling of all the women who never really knew the ''right'' thing to wear or couldn't afford it anyway even if they did know what was ''right.''

The Georgetown ladies in their Halstons, their boots, and their fashionably straight hair sneered at Rosalynn. That is, the ladies in the boots, the Halstons, and the short hair sneered, until Rosalynn became First Lady. Then wash-and-wear became acceptable, if not reverse chic. Inaugural tales flew about Washington ladies from Georgia in Tammy Wynette hairdos and gentlemen from Alabama in their tuxedos and brown shoes. All the sneering was for nought. Winners can afford to be out of style.

Or at least winners who live in the White House. The fashion industry weighed the pros and cons of Rosalynn's out-of-style dress. Women's editors debated the fact that Betty Ford patronized American designers and Rosalynn shopped in Americus, Georgia. Over and over, writers lauded Rosalynn's practical style of dressing. Well, she lived in the White House and that made her strange tastes respectable.

However most people want to be in style because *au courant* dress indicates success and shows to the world that you are part of the well-heeled cognoscenti. Not only do you dress in the current fashion—but you can be first (or second) to wear boots, gaucho pants, three-piece men's suits, or whatever. Moreover, by being *au courant* you advertise to the world your own financial stability—or that of your husband. Dress, style, physical appearance, and demeanor are proclamations of a certain station in life. For a supposedly classless society, we have enough status symbols to make the Egyptians look like amateurs.

For example, straight teeth imply good breeding. Or good orthodontia. Or a doting father with lots of money to spend on his children's teeth. Not only teeth, but nearly every aspect of physical appearance itself is a reflection of social class and money. Good prenatal care, adequate obstetrical services, clean hospitals, and a high protein diet ensure the middle class of children who are straight of limb and back. When a middle-class child is born with some infirmity, thousands of dollars are spent to rid the child of whatever curse has befallen. Yet even though physical appearance is basic to our innermost care values, most people are unable to admit that they cannot tolerate misshapen bodies or scarred faces.

I used to make my students in a class on marriage and the family list those characteristics they wanted in a husband or wife. Sometimes students would say "pretty" or "handsome," but mostly they listed pitiful clichés like "successful," "well-rounded," "good personality," or "good education." Then I would ask them to list the characteristics they did *not* want in a husband or wife. Some of the honest students admitted that they would not marry a person of a different race or religion but, again, most listed trite answers. Not one student in over ten years of teaching this course ever said, "I would not marry a blind girl," or "I would not marry a crippled man."

That's probably because blind, deaf, halt, or disfigured boys and girls just aren't in their circle of friends. At a very early age, blind, deaf, and crippled students are sent to special schools which cater to their very special problems. While there is indeed a humanitarian aspect to special training for the handicapped, special schools are dumping grounds so that the "normal" students will not have to associate with the "abnormal." Those with garden-variety disfigurements like birthmarks or a hare lip are in for a life of calvary, beginning with grade school. Children are so very cruel.

"Sticks and stones can break my bones and names will break my psyche." I shudder on remembering how nasty I was to those boys and girls in grade school who had to wear glasses. "Four Eyes" was the very least epithet we hurled at the weak-eyed yokums of the fifth grade. "Fatso," "Two-Ton," and "Blimpo" are yelled out every day at every recess period throughout the United States. Children start off early learning that people who look a little odd are fair game.

Teachers don't help either. Recent studies indicate that if you want to guarantee your child's success in school make sure that he or she is neatly dressed and clean. Teachers spend more time with clean children than dirty children. It is psychologically understandable but educationally reprehensible that a teacher spends more time with Alice-in-Wonderland with the red pinafore than with Maria Gonzalez in her shabby patched cotton dress.

A handsome or pretty child soon learns to capitalize on his or her good looks. My aunt and uncle tell a tale of woe concerning one of my cousins. Throughout grade school at the PTA meetings my cousin Peter's teachers would gush to Aunt Florence, "My, Peter is such a lovely child. My, he is a lovely student. And those eyelashes! I have never seen eyelashes like that on a boy ever in my whole life!" It was true. Peter had the longest, silkiest, and most gorgeous eyelashes of anyone in our family. When he lowered his eyes, it looked as though he had silky black fans resting on his cheeks. However, all those teachers who gushed over Peter's manners and good grades were women. In grade seven, Peter got a male teacher. The story was considerably different on grade seven PTA night. Aunt Florence learned that Peter was really not too well mannered and his grades needed a great deal of improvement. The male teacher was not impressed by Peter's eyelashes at all.

I include this vignette to illustrate that men can play the sex-beauty game as well as women. One reason why I have always been suspicious of good-looking men is that they are invariably arrogant. Like my handsome cousin, Peter, attractive-looking men receive adulation from women teachers, adoring female relatives, slathering sorority girls, and slavish secretaries. A truly handsome six-foot-four Greek god commands attention and demands obedience. For example, the army talks about "command presence." In other words, the Pentagon seems to choose generals who look like Hollywood thinks generals should look. Tall and sinewy of frame, bold of chin, flinty of eye—a general should have command presence. Which probably explains why service academies used to have a minimum-height requirement. Napoleon notwithstanding, who could respect a little teeny general? Well, that question may be answered in the year 2000 when short men and tiny women become the generals of that era.

Lady generals aside, a combination of beauty-brains can be fatal for women. A friend of mine once sat in on an admission board of a large medical school. One of the applicants was a highly qualified young woman with excellent grades and superior recommendations. However, she was also a slender, green-eyed, stunning brunette with a creamy complexion. The august members of the medical school refused her admittance on the grounds that she would be a disturbing influence on her fellow male students. My friend, who is a lady psychiatrist, threw a temper tantrum. She demanded that her colleagues rethink their own psychological reactions to this young woman. When the male board members finally saw that they were reacting sexually and not intellectually to the beautiful young applicant, they reversed their decision.

Sometimes a reverse stereotype persists. Women who work in male occupations must perforce be ugly. Lady truck drivers, lady mechanics, lady construction workers, lady cops are really not ladies. But they are. These women have chosen these occupations because they wanted to be officers, or construction workers, or mechanics, or lawyers. Also these women wanted the high salaries associated with these occupations. One interesting TV news interview with two women coal miners involved the question of how you could be feminine and a coal miner. Both women were reasonably inarticulate, but their replies were penetrating. They both said that they didn't want to be women in a man's occupation but they were tired of earning low salaries above ground, and they were going to work below ground for high union salaries. No women's liberation for them; just equality of a paycheck.

I am sure that lady coal miners change clothes and take baths and put on dresses after work, just as lady cops do. Slowly—and admittedly, thanks to the mass media—there is a new message coming across to the American public. Women do not have to sacrifice "femininity" to work in men's jobs.

The question then arises, what exactly is "femininity"? Or whose standards of femininity do we use? Does "feminine" mean being a simpering, passive little ninny with flouncy, bouncy curls and fluttering eyelashes? Do you have to stop dressing in a pretty or, if you will, feminine manner in order to succeed in business? These really are burning issues even though they seem at first glance to be relatively ephemeral. Some young girls think that they have to become man-hating, ugly witches if they want to become doctors or lawyers. As a consequence, these young women who may have brains and ability do *not* become doctors or lawyers. Thus talented people (who happen to be women) are wasted in trivial, low-level jobs, simply because they listened to some silly stereotypes.

These misconceptions are alive and well and fostered by the mass media and anti-ERA forces. Groups like Fascinating Womanhood or Phyllis Schlafly's followers contend that all a woman has to do is be a good wife and mother in order to fulfill her obligation to society at large. Wifeness and motherhood are important, but they are not all inclusive. You can be wife and mother and working woman and pretty and feminine. It is hard, but it can be done. The heartening fact is that there are some chic, sleek, brainy, and very feminine women who think that makeup and pretty clothes are not inimical to brains and high salaries.

I am always amazed when people meet women cadets from West Point, Annapolis, or the Air Force Academy. The first comment is usually, "But you're so pretty!" Then the next quip is, "Why is a nice girl like you in a service academy!" The reply is, of course, "Why not?" So now style sections of Sunday magazines feature pretty women who work in male jobs. Rosie the Riveter has returned in a new guise. A new chic has arrived.

However, the protagonists are different. West Point women, women medical students, female M.B.S.'s, and lady Ph.D.'s are a new breed of cat. Or at least they seem to be more relaxed than a generation ago. The current generation grew up in blue jeans through grade school, high school, and undergraduate years with only a few forays to occasional dress-up occasions. They are probably less enslaved by the wild seesawing of Parisian couturiers than the over-forty crowd. They realize that clothes are meant to be fun and comfortable. As a matter of fact, the over-forty crowd has a lot to learn about relaxing and hanging loose. If you observe different age women in the same social situation, differences are incredibly marked.

For example, after dinner in a restaurant, forty-year-olds usually dash to the ladies' room or frantically put on their lipstick at the table. It's almost as though not having lipstick on is the equivalent of being nude in public. Under-thirty women sometimes put on lipstick, but usually ignore the ritual. The in-betweeners, the thirties, are divided on their reaction. But even though makeup seems to be less important to the new woman, booming cosmetic sales belie that fact. Yet we should remember that the baby-boom girls are now thirty-year-olds fighting crow's-feet and bags under the eyes. Many of these women are also fighting loneliness, depression, inflation, and recalcitrant teen-agers.

For it's not only wrinkles in the hard light of a winter's morning looking into the bathroom mirror that are frightening, but a dream gone sour. *Modern Bride*'s vision, *McCall*'s message, *Cosmo*'s hype, and *True Confession*'s advice just don't work out. One out of every three marriages in the United States ends up in divorce, and in some areas, one out of every two. And that's the basic fear of most women. *He* will walk out. You'll never see *him* again. *He* won't pay the bills anymore. *He* won't support the children. You will be alone. And it often happens.

The media constantly tell American women how to dress, look, act, perform sexually, and cook delightfully. Step by step we are told how to attract, snare, entrap, and hopefully keep a man. But it's the keeping part that's so hard. Since youth is attractive, every passing year means that you are less attractive, unless you use a certain cream or emollient. Even then there's no guarantee that he will stick around, unless you learn some interesting gymnastics, courtesy of Alex Comfort or "Tell Me, Doctor" columns.

What happens when he walks out? Therein lies another tale. The media spare no details on how a man is necessary to a woman's survival. The over-forty-year-old who is suddenly abandoned is grist for many an editorial. These women are held up as dire examples of women who "let themselves go." The message here is that the man walked out because he found someone else more attractive. If Mary Middle-aged had only used such and such a cream or didn't have a smelly refrigerator, her husband would still be in her nice warm bed. Maybe.

The media are responding sympathetically to these late-divorce women. Magazines and newspapers feature the pain of an abandoned woman—regardless of her social class. It sells papers. But more important for the future of women in this country, magazines in particular show how women *must* have skills to support themselves in case divorce occurs. It *is* damned hard to be the divorced or widowed mother of two teen-agers, hold down a job, cook, clean, shop, and hold on to one's sanity. Yet it is better to be employed than unemployed and it is better to have a white-collar well-paying job than a low-paying job. It seems at first glance to be reasonable, economic, and sociological sense, but most girls have never heard that message and suffer when they are older women. So at least in this instance, magazines are responding in a sensible manner to a severe social problem. Soap operas still emphasize the need for a woman to catch a man—the second or third time. Soap heroines are never self-reliant.

Magazines are more sensitive to the "new woman" or her "problems" because the magazine industry is slowly sinking into a morass of bankruptcy. Magazines have to respond to a fickle audience in order to maintain their advertisers and stay in business. Thus magazines have reacted and responded to radical feminist critiques, some serious self-criticisms by women journalists, and in rare instances visionary leadership by women editors. Some *True Confession* stories show women as decisive actors rather than poor, downtrodden victims. Sometimes the blue-collar magazines even advocate outright militancy in regard to equal pay. Middle-class magazines like *McCall's* and *Ladies' Home Journal* have caught on to the fact that women are working. Interestingly enough, the fact that women are working, are earning their own salaries, are mistresses of their own destiny, and are making their own financial decisions has had the most impact on magazines. Women's liberation is now O.K. Women are not necessarily all dummies. As a result of the media becoming aware that women are indeed better informed and more alert, new editorial policies have been promulgated. In particular we see that middle-class magazines now feature more and more articles dealing with "female" medicine.

Thanks to Betty Ford's honesty and the publicity surrounding Happy Rockefeller's mastectomy, women's magazines discuss breast cancer. Well aware that women in the United States view mastectomy with horror, these magazines do perform a viable and worthwhile public service in discussing what previously was a taboo topic. The magazine articles point out that losing a mass of muscle is preferable to losing one's life. Going against the prevalent media message that perfection of body is equated with happiness, these articles show that a mastectomy is not the end of the world. Magazine editors found out that the groundswell of interest and sympathy surrounding Mrs. Ford's and Mrs. Rockefeller's operations meant that American women desperately needed information and reassurance. To their credit, the magazines responded in an adult and responsible fashion. Young women journalists have also launched an attack on the differential treatment women receive from their male gynecologists and general practitioners.

Following the lead of Barbara Seaman, writers now ask why there are more mastectomies and hysterectomies in the United States than in Europe or England. *McCall's* and *Ladies' Home Journal* in particular have detailed discussion of alternatives to radical mastectomies. These writers show that women can have lumps aspirated before a breast operation is performed. If the lump is cancerous, maybe only a partial resection is necessary rather than the enormous radical surgery performed by United States doctors.

Magazines now debate other topics like the danger of the birth-control pill, complications in using an intrauterine device, pills during pregnancy, and the pros and cons of abortion. Thanks to the women's magazines, American women are becoming more and more aware of the kinds of questions that they ought to ask their doctors. Rather than fostering passive acceptance, many articles in the middle-class magazines encourage questioning demands.

Just as we see that not all magazine writers are tools of a Madison Avenue conspiracy, soap operas are slowly edging into the twentieth century. One soap opera, *The Young and the Restless*, showed how a rape victim became the subject of innuendo during the subsequent trial. *The Young and the Restless* also portrayed the psychological problems a woman encountered after having a mastectomy. Mass media have found that their audience are not stupid and are eager for intelligent information.

Women social scientists, on the other hand, have learned that they can use mass-media styles to reach a wide audience. Marjorie Ford Crow and Felicia Guest, both health educators in the Emory University School of Medicine Family Planning Program, noted that lower-class women were involved in and affected by true-confession magazines. Crow and Guest wrote pamphlets in the same breathless pulp manner exhorting women to take control of their own fertility. Derided by their colleagues and praised by the American College of Obstetricians and Gynecologists, Crow and Guest have found an effective method of communicating to a hitherto estranged group.

But these are only a few faint glimmers. Even though women become more aware of Madison Avenue's machinations, they still accept advertising's fake standards. Cleanliness is not only next to but really *is* godliness. A woman who has waxy buildup on her kitchen floor is worse than someone who has pins in her bra straps.

Women receive a new, impossible message. Work and be fulfilled! Take your salary and buy these labor-saving devices. Crock-pots. Instant coffee. Instant potatoes. Dehydrated soups. Super bubbling and humming cleanser! Zigzag sewing machines. Wash and wax and vacuum cleaners. Dicer-slicers. All these wonderful products will save you time and make your life better. Not only will you whiz through your household chores, but you will become a gracious hostess. But it never really works out that way. Home economics professors point out that the more labor-saving devices we have in the home, the more time women spend using them.

Demands for cleanliness reach absurd heights and show how we can become enslaved to our machines. I remember the days of washer-wringers and outdoor clotheslines. That meant that my mother did one load or two of washing on a specific day and that towels had to last for a week. Even when I went to college, the dormitory gave us only one set of towels per week. Enter washers with spin dryers and washing became "easier." But it really wasn't easier because Tide and Cheer added to our household burdens. Jingles and refrains screamed the sin of "ring around the collar'' and "tattle-tale gray.'' Commercials became miniature soap operas with distraught housewives bewailing the fact that their colors were not bright enough or whites not white enough. Hours were added to household work. The new message, courtesy of new machines and magic soaps, said that we should have clean towels *every* day.

That of course explained why my sister-in-law, Leona, spent most of her waking hours in a dank basement. A doctor's wife with a luxurious mansion, Leona believed that her role as housewife meant that her family must have clean clothes and fluffy towels at all times. She ran up and down steps to her washer and dryer, washing, drying, folding, sorting, and fulfilling her role as good *Hausfrau*. The problem was, though, that Leona's family saw very little of her except in her forays up and down the stairs. When I asked her once, "Why do you constantly wash every day—day and night?" She replied, "Migod, my family needs clean towels." I tried to explain that her family needed *her*. Shortly after that she entered therapy. She still does a lot of washing. Poor Leona, she really believed that being a good wife and mother was equated with housework, or that it was solely and exclusively equated with housework.

Most of us are like Leona. We accede to impossible standards of cleanliness because copywriters know how to prey on a woman's sense of guilt. Just watch television one afternoon or in the early evening and see how insidious and ingenious these messages really are.

Yellow kitchen floors tell the world that Harriet

Housewife is incompetent. Use Mop & Glo and orgiastic delights will follow. I used Mop & Glo and my sex life was still lousy. Smart lady plumbers use Drano, while stupid housewives don't. Lemon Fresh Joy makes your dishes shine and your relatives marvel at your housewifery. Duncan Hines cakes are better than homemade. The list is endless. Promises eternal. Perfection is obtained on your grocer's shelves. Perfection, cleanliness, godliness, gracious hospitality, and an adoring family are attained through the purchase of Lemon Fresh Joy and Drano.

Quite obviously not all of us believe that message. Yet most of us *want* the promises to come true. Why not? Maybe Geritol or Clairol will produce a new me and a more rapturous spouse. Maybe a Toni permanent will produce more orgasms. Anyway, it's worth the gamble of a few dollars.

So fashion and the media message go on. Soap-opera messages are interspersed with soap advertising. They all get mixed up in some weird Kafka mishmash. Periodically it's worthwhile to stand back from the boutique-grocery-hairdresser phase and ask yourself what exactly you are doing and why. If you can answer honestly about your dreams and fears, your beauty quest is reasonably healthy.

And if the answers are dishonest, hold on to the dream.

Sources

1. Carbohydrate Counters is a not-so-fictitious organization whose description is based on participant observation and membership in a nationally franchised weight-reducing club, observation of a locally organized diet club, and interviews with lecturers and members of three different diet clubs in five different states. In addition, four sister social scientists who have belonged in four separate states to a nationally franchised diet club have relayed their impressions to me. For a discussion of an independent diet club see Natalie Allon, "Group Dieting Interaction," unpublished Ph.D. dissertation, Brandeis University, 1972. For an analysis of a local diet club in Cleveland in the mid-1950's see Marvin Sussman, "The Calorie Collectors: A Study of Spontaneous Group Formation, Collapse and Reconstruction," *Social Forces*, **34** (May, 1956 (a)): 351-56, and

"Psycho-Social Correlates of Obesity: Failure of 'Calorie Collectors,' " *Journal of the American Dietetic Association,* **32** (May, 1956 (b)): 425-28. Peter Wyden, *The Overweight Society* (New York: William Morrow and Co., 1965), chapter 5, discusses TOPS (Take Off Pounds Sensibly). Articles and books dealing with Weight Watchers, Inc., include Jean Nidetch, *The Story of Weight Watchers* (New York: New American Library, 1970); Kathrin Perutz, *Beyond the Looking Glass: America's Beauty Culture* (New York: William Morrow and Co., 1970), pp. 165-70; *Time,* February 21, 1972: 71-72; "Fortune from Fat," *Vogue,* **151** (Jan. 21, 1968): 34. An organization similar to Jean Nidetch's Weight Watchers, which also was patterned on the Morrisania clinic of Dr. Norman Jolliffe, is Diet Watchers, described in Ann Gold and Sara Wells Briller, *Diet Watcher's Guide* (New York: Grosset and Dunlap, 1968); and a comparable Indianapolis organization, Weightless Wonders, is the subject of an *Indianapolis Star Magazine* article, November 2, 1969, entitled, "TLC for Dieters," by L. A. Stauffer.

2. Norman Jolliffe, *Reduce and Stay Reduced* (New York: Simon and Schuster, 1952); Norman Jolliffe and Morton B. Glenn, "Obesity," in Norman Jolliffe, ed., *Clinical Nutrition* (New York: Harper & Row, 1962), pp. 820-90.

3. Richard Aronson and Richard Epstein, *The Miracle of Cosmetic Plastic Surgery* (Los Angeles: Sherborne Press, 1970); William Brown, *Cosmetic Surgery* (New York: Stein and Day, 1970); Simona Morina, *Body Sculpture: Surgery from Head to Toe* (New York: Delacorte Press, 1972); Thomas Ress and Donald Wood-Smith, *Cosmetic Facial Surgery* (Philadelphia: Saunders, 1973); James W. Smith and Samm Sinclair Baker, *"Doctor, Make Me Beautiful!"* (New York: McKay, 1973); Kurt Wagner and Helen

Gould, *How to Win in the Youth Game: The Magic of Plastic Surgery* (Englewood Cliffs, N.J.: Prentice-Hall, 1972).

4. Caroline Isber and Muriel Canter, *Report of the Task Force on Women in Public Broadcasting*, Corporation for Public Broadcasting, Washington, D.C., 1975.

Index